MANAGEMENT
360 Degrees

'Basant Chaudhary provides an illuminating perspective on a wide range of topical areas which are of great relevance to business leaders, individuals and the wider regions and communities. While adopting an introspective and detailed approach, Mr Chaudhary offers contextual solutions in an array of different business and social environments. His insightful and objective viewpoint on relevant and thought-provoking subjects, and wise words are meaningful contributions to the discourse on the challenges and realities facing Nepal and the world, today and tomorrow.'

—**Prof. Gaven R. R. Caldwell**
Chief Executive Officer,
International Management Institute, Switzerland

'It makes me happy that Basant Chaudhary is sharing his business and management experiences and knowledge with the world at large through *Management 360 Degrees*. It is this sharing attitude that has earned him respect and admiration from people at large over the years. The book is indeed worth more than one read.'

—**Binod Chaudhary**
Member of the Parliament of Nepal and Chairperson,
Chaudhary Group

MANAGEMENT
360 Degrees

Making a New Nepal

BASANT CHAUDHARY

RUPA

Published by
Rupa Publications India Pvt. Ltd 2023
7/16, Ansari Road, Daryaganj
New Delhi 110002

Sales Centres:
Prayagraj Bengaluru Chennai
Hyderabad Jaipur Kathmandu
Kolkata Mumbai

P-ISBN: 978-93-5520-760-9
E-ISBN: 978-93-5520-762-3

First impression 2023

10 9 8 7 6 5 4 2 3 1

Printed in India

Contents

Foreword

In recent years policymakers and planners have been emphasizing on the role of good institutions as prerequisite for building a nation. An institution needs good management to effectively deliver results for which it is established. It is well accepted now that of all the resources available in a country, management is the one whose quality alone can determine the extent of utilization of resources. Peter F. Drucker, the giant of management philosophy, once observed that a country is underdeveloped because it is undermanaged. For a poor country like Nepal where every bit of resource needs to be carefully utilized, the significance of good management cannot be undermined. The poor performance of our economy is due to our failure to manage our institutions effectively and efficiently. Management has become a critical constraint for the development of Nepal.

One way to make people aware of the importance of management is to initiate and encourage dialogue about the management practices, culture, values and philosophies. The value of Western management culture and practices are indeed important for us to understand the way institutions are managed. However, we should understand that management is also an attitude and culture. What we observe and learn from the Western management practices and styles cannot be copied as they are meant to solve our problems without modifying our culture and needs. This poses a big challenge in a system like ours—closed, cynical, and non-transparent.

Basant Chaudhary, who has been at the helm of diversified businesses in manufacturing and services for over four decades, has initiated laudable efforts to share his experience with the general public at large, particularly with the youths who need good advice and guidance to enter and run business. As a seasoned businessman who knows the ins and outs of the business system of Nepal, Chaudhary has provided extremely valuable and practical suggestions through a series of write-ups published in *Business 360* under the 'Business Sutra' column. In a country like Nepal where a majority of businessmen avoid sharing their experiences and keep their business closely guarded, Chaudhary has made an important contribution in the arena of management in Nepal by sharing his experience and knowledge.

In this book *Management 360 Degrees: Making a New Nepal* the author has touched upon diverse areas of management and addressed important issues in contemporary business and management in Nepal. He expresses his concern over gender issues and emphasizes on the role of women, and pleads for providing women with legitimate opportunity while also providing tips for their success. He deals with the issues in leadership and values, and discusses the Confucian way to grand success and the importance of yoga for business. He focuses on Business Dharma and expresses concern over the breeding greed in business. He talks about Steve Job's emphasis on quality, Narayan Murty's 'gyan', Warren Buffet's strategy, Indira Nooyi as the 'Cola Lady' and other management leaders. His narration about the operation of Mumbai's dabbawalas (tiffin service operators) reveals the importance of system efficiency and quality monitoring of the service.

On contemporary issues Chaudhary expresses his concern over environment and climate change and draws our attention towards artificial intelligence and the need to leverage social media. His write-ups also deal with several practical problems facing an organization, like office politics, corporate burnouts, emotional pressure points, self-management, response to feedback, etc. He suggests ways to deal with an overbearing boss. He emphasizes on the importance of communication and suggests ways to deal with change. Some of his write-ups also deal with entrepreneurship and intra-prenuership. He expresses his concern over the condition of management education and emphasizes on the need to make it more practical and close to business reality.

Unlike most businessmen who tend to be engrossed in their business solely and wholly, B.K. Chaudhary's write-ups highlight his continuous zeal to keep himself abreast of what is going around in business and academia. He cites reports of the Harvard Business Review, International Monetary Fund, and World Bank, apart from drawing key learnings from various conferences, in his write-ups. Using a simple and easy-to-understand language, Chaudhary has managed to share his views in a persuasive and convincing manner, even though at times one does get the impression that the author got carried away with the flow of his thoughts.

This book is a valuable contribution in the field of management in Nepal and will be fruitful to those who are eager to know about management practices. *Management 360 Degrees: Making a New Nepal* is unique as it narrates the experiences and learnings of a stalwart in business and management in Nepal.

Prof. Bijay K.C.
Dean, Kathmandu University School of Management

Introduction

I started writing regularly on issues and events related to Nepal in 2015 and the catalyst for doing so was an earthquake—probably the most disastrous in living memory—that claimed the lives of more than 8,000 people. The damage to the nation's psyche was even more than the losses in property and infrastructure. Nepal's growth and development were set back by at least a decade. Till date, industries and businesses are yet to fully recover from that shock.

It was in this backdrop that I started looking towards the future with the hope of rebuilding Nepal. I quickly realized the urgent need for communicating with young Nepalese managers and executives on ways to work towards developing Nepal rapidly. I started sharing my views on the economy, geopolitics and business management through articles in newspapers and magazines. The response encouraged me to sharpen my focus and dwell mainly on the latest skills, tools and other developments related to management. As was my intention, young people soon outnumbered others as my readers.

Having been at the helm of a diversified business conglomerate with footprints in both manufacturing and services, I strongly felt that Nepal's future lay in strengthening its industrial and business landscape. For this, young entrants in the corporate world needed experience-based mentoring by seasoned practitioners. By 2016, the sundry articles were transformed into a regular column in Nepal's reputed business monthly *Business 360°*. 'Business Sutra', the column, continues to be published in multiple editions of the magazine till date. My business experience of over four decades is now in your hands in the form of this volume—a compilation of some the best columns authored by me.

People of Nepal also know me for my lyrical compositions in Nepali, Hindi and Urdu that still form the bulk of my literary oeuvre. Much before I started writing, my poems were available in the form of books and music discs, and were received well by the critics and the masses, in general. Even though my love affair with poetry continues unabated, I have authored two books on contemporary issues confronting Nepal, and *Management 360 Degrees: Making a New Nepal* is part of my continued efforts to create the Nepal of our dreams. This collection is also significant because it documents the tumultuous events and changes that took place during a very critical phase of transition in Nepal's history.

The practice and teaching of business management is a highly dynamic process. For sheer survival, today's businesses need to continually reinvent and renew themselves. While some management theories continue to hold fort, new postulations, methodologies, skills and tools keep on making their appearance with surprising regularity. They are tested on the touchstone of business reality, and depending upon their applicability, some of them are absorbed, while others are discarded.

Of late, modifications in management practice have been dictated by technology that has become synonymous with change. Change is easier to spell but difficult to implement. Technological change creates new templates that demand behavioural change. Humans are not easily amenable to altering their ways. Managers, young and old, have to meet the challenge of adapting to the changing management practices. The trouble is that business schools, more so in my part of the world, have only a fragile link with the real needs of the business sector. Education remains largely academic in nature. It is, therefore, incumbent upon promoters and senior practitioners of management to share their experiences and wisdom with management students and fresh entrants within the business world in whichever way they can. It cannot be a one-off measure. Mentoring and tempering should be an ever-flowing river. After all, flowing water remains fresh.

It has been my endeavour to upskill young corporate citizens through my columns. The world they are facing today is far more competitive than in our times, when we started our entrepreneurial journey. At the same time, young managers are fortunate to be able to access information and knowledge far more rapidly, thanks to the ever-happening advances in technology. Are our youngsters willing to march to the drumbeat? Are they ready to switch over to the new beats? But most importantly, are they good enough to create their own rhythm, one in sync with their national ethos, culture and resource base? There is no need to be overwhelmed by the spate of management offerings, many of which are mere fads. Pick and choose with wisdom, keeping the fluff apart. I hope that *Management 360 Degrees: Making a New Nepal* helps you in making that informed decision.

My sincere appreciation goes to Charu Chaddha, editor of *Business 360°*, who gave me an opportunity to write for her prestigious magazine. Similarly, a big thanks goes to Dibakar Ghosh of Rupa Publications for finding this book suitable for publication. My special thanks go to Shreepa Shrestha and Saluja Shrestha for helping me complete my book. Without them, it would not have been possible to publish this. The most important person in this has been my dear daughter, Megha Chaudhary, who is also the foremost critic of my writings. She continues to help me with writing ideas and is always there to inspire me.

The Glass Ceiling

March 2016

There are several facts of life we are all well aware of. Yet we choose to overlook them. One of them is gender discrimination. The deeply entrenched patriarchal system in our society has been denying women their due for ages. Despite possessing the required qualifications, competencies and abilities, women find themselves lagging behind their equally or even less proficient male counterparts in most professions. The problem is not restricted to the less developed countries as is generally believed. Women professionals bear the brunt of this discrimination even in the most advanced countries.

The corporate world which swears by meritocracy and thrives on performance-based efficiency too is a guilty party of this malaise. Women fail to rise beyond a point and the top positions and boardrooms are packed with men.

This is what has come to be known as the 'glass ceiling'. It is invisible. Yet it takes tremendous effort for women corporate executives to break it and move up in the organizational hierarchy. Many women have managed to do that. But they are exceptions considering their large and growing number in the corporate sector.

Former editor of *Working Woman* Gay Bryant was quoted in an *Adweek* interview in the 1980s as saying, 'Women have reached a certain point—I call it the glass ceiling. They're in the top of middle management and they're stopping and getting stuck. There isn't enough room for all those women at the top. Some are going into business for themselves. Others are going out and raising families.' *The Wall Street Journal* carried an article in March 1986 headlined *The Glass Ceiling: Why Women Can't Seem to Break the Invisible Barrier that Blocks Them from the Top Jobs.*

The debate has gained momentum since then. In 1991, the US Labor Department's research project called 'Glass Ceiling Initiative' defined the new term as 'those artificial barriers based on attitudinal or organizational bias that prevent qualified individuals from advancing upward in their organization into management-level positions'. (This report had, however, also covered discrimination based on ethnicity.)

This is despite the fact that today's private companies are competing in a global environment and need the best available and affordable talent to survive and grow. Preventing our competent female managers and executives from attaining their full potential can be suicidal for companies. Also, this will deter girls from joining the corporate workforce.

Noted management and HRD expert Dr Hema Krishnan, currently Professor of Strategic Management in Xavier University, Ohio, USA, has made some highly significant observations: (a) having an increased representation of women in top positions sends a positive signal to the rest of the organization and augurs well for the treatment of other women; (b) a woman's leadership style, often perceived to be nurturing, inspires confidence among her peers and subordinates, and especially among other women; and (c) women play multiple roles in their personal lives, which sharpens their interpersonal, conflict resolution and other leadership skills. This combination of adaptability, interaction with peers and subordinates, and an ability to nurture and inspire can help an organization to succeed.

Yet progression to the top management remains a major challenge for most aspiring and deserving women managers. What is the way out?

The first step involves identifying the key competencies within your company and then assessing how much you are aligned with them. This is called core competence analysis. While a conservative company will value employees who are analytical, careful and avoid risks, another, focused on innovation, will prefer risk takers who express themselves openly. You will thus find yourself tied closely to the respective company's culture and vision. You will have a good understanding of the attributes of the organization's top management. Chances of promotion will rise.

So far so good! Now move beyond understanding of the targets. Set goals to get there. (You can consult your reporting authority.) This is personal goal setting. Take the initiative. Do not wait for tasks to be handed over to you. You should let your boss know that you are willing to go the extra mile and take on additional responsibilities. Seek his/her advice about new skills you need to learn. It is essential to keep on monitoring and measuring your progress.

Compared to their male colleagues, women managers are known for paying less attention to professional networking. This can and does affect their career growth. It is essential to build relationships at all levels in the organization not only for ease of work but also for information gathering. Building ties only with the top management is not the best idea. It may alienate you from your peers. You need all your skills to rise to the top and stay there. Meet newcomers regularly. Get involved with cross-functional teams. Your professional networking should extend outside of your organization too. Do not forget that in case you fail to break the glass ceiling in your own organization, then you may need to look for options outside.

A mentor can be the best conduit to upward growth. The mentor is usually a senior person in top management. He/She has an inside view of the company's thought process at the highest decision-making level. He/She can prove to be a reliable source of information and also help you in making sense of the information. Given his/her experience, you can expect invaluable professional tips from such a person. It is best to seek mentoring support from your immediate boss and then move upwards.

It is equally important to ensure that you develop your competence, leadership skills, communication skills, technical know-how and other competencies that people at the top expect from potential fast trackers. While your eyes are set on the top management, those at the helm are also always looking for mid-level managers who can be promoted to the organization's executive committees, board of directors, etc. Are you visible to them from the top? Have you been seeking and excelling in high-profile projects? Have you been making vital and practical contributions in meetings? That is, have you been able to build a reputation for yourself? Try to create one in areas where you are lacking so that you are easily identifiable as top management material.

As you are planning to rise to the top by breaking the invisible glass ceiling it is obvious that you should be ready to face and fight discriminatory behaviour if any. Gender-based biases, prejudices and stereotypes have deep roots in our society. Besides competence and other abilities you will need a lot of grit and perseverance to tackle this challenge. Emotional intelligence plays a vital role here. Knowledge of your rights, company policies and local laws is essential too.

I look forward to more and more deserving women finding their rightful place in top corporate management.

Change, But Communicate

April 2016

Is it possible to do nothing wrong and yet lose? Seems unlikely? But it happens. It has happened, again and again. Many companies are realizing this now. Alas, it is too late for some of them!

The globalized and competitive market is merciless. It has its own dynamics. Those averse to change and communication perish. Those who are able to read the writing on the wall and embrace change flourish. For some reason, a heart-rending speech of Nokia's then CEO is doing the rounds of social media currently. Speaking at a press conference to announce Nokia's acquisition by Microsoft, Nokia's CEO said in a choked voice, 'We didn't do anything wrong, but somehow, we lost.' That was the worst hour of grief and mourning for the world's one-time largest cell phone maker.

Nokia had overtaken Motorola to reach the top spot in 1998. Samsung had just entered the market then and was struggling. Nokia controlled around 40 per cent of the market for years till Apple Inc. came out with its iPhone in 2007. Apple's revolutionary product soon overtook Nokia's smartphones. Nokia felt compelled to tie up with Microsoft in 2011 to use its Windows phone platform. September

2013 witnessed Microsoft announcing its resolve to acquire Nokia's mobile business as part of an overall deal worth $7.17 billion. Stephen Elop, Nokia's former CEO, and several other executives joined the new Microsoft mobile subsidiary of Microsoft as part of the deal, which was completed on 25 April 2014.

Oh, how the mighty fall! But they do leave lessons for the top brass and business managers. Management leaders and gurus have racked their brains to analyse and understand the fall of the giant Finnish MNC. In a nutshell, the inference is that Nokia refused to acknowledge the power of change and the need for communication. Its mindset remained frozen. Nokia lost in the race for survival. The competitors seized the opportunity to race ahead and make the one-time leader extinct.

In his bestseller *The 7 Habits of Highly Effective People*, Stephen Covey highlighted the dire need for reinventing oneself regularly in five realms, namely, physical, social, emotional, mental and spiritual. Only then can one meet new challenges which spring suddenly out of nowhere.

Experts have pointed out time and again that a company's current competitive advantage cannot last forever, especially if it ignores new technology, management ethos, trends and customer needs. So, even without doing anything 'wrong' you can lose if you refuse to do the right thing at the right time.

Businesses operating within relatively protected environments like Nepal also need to gauge the way the wind is blowing. You cannot beat the onward march of technology. You cannot beat modern and proactive modes of management by sticking to a feudal business mindset and refusing to communicate with your stakeholders.

Entrepreneurs are on the rise everywhere. They are the real green shoots for an underdeveloped economy like ours. Only they seem to have the potential to grow into mighty oaks. Reason: entrepreneurs and progressive businesses respect change and follow its pace. They are nimble-footed and do not carry the baggage of worn-out business systems which are still dependent on political and official patronage, centralized decision-making and nepotism.

Getting back to the reasons adduced by experts for the fall of big corporations let me return to Nokia and then cite some other significant examples. Complacency has been found to be one of the major causes of the terminal decline of companies. Nokia kept its eyes virtually closed to Apple's launch of the iPhone, the first touch phone, in 2007. Samsung, on the other hand, launched its smartphones using off-the-shelf technologies.

Nokia ignored innovation at its own peril. Samsung has been coming up with new phone models frequently, though with slight upgrades only. Nokia's Window phone, launched in 2011, lacked some basic technology. Its Lumia series too failed to attract trendy youngsters. It did not even have a front camera. That means it was not even 3G enabled. Clearly, Nokia had failed to prepare for the future. No wonder, then, that the future failed Nokia.

But writing in the *Harvard Business Review (HBR)* Michael Schrage, a Research Fellow at the MIT Sloan School of Management's Initiative on the Digital Economy, refused to believe that Nokia had lost its ability to innovate. He asserted, 'There's a simpler and more strategic explanation for why this once-perennial market leader became second-rate. Nokia ignored America. The company simply refused to compete energetically, ingeniously and respectfully in the U.S. America was treated as an innovation afterthought. Nokia tried to get away with preserving its market dominance in Europe and growing its leadership in Asia. The richest country in the world was, literally and figuratively, a third-class priority for the Finnish giant... Marginalizing America allowed two of Nokia's most dangerous competitors to swiftly, safely, and smartly out-innovate it.' A massive strategic miscalculation, indeed!

Another article in *HBR* in 2012 by Boris Groysberg, professor of Business Administration at Harvard Business School, and Michael Slind, communications consultant, found poor communication as the main reason for corporate disasters, including the one that struck Nokia. According to the duo, Nokia lost its competitive edge because of 'habits of communication that favor(ed) unfocused discussions about strategy over clear plans to bring new phone models to market.'

US energy giant Enron collapsed because of 'communication-based leader responsibilities' that senior managers failed to meet—responsibilities such as 'communicating appropriate values' and 'maintaining openness to signs of problems.'

The blowout of the Deepwater Horizon offshore oil rig in April 2010 resulted in a massive crisis for BP (formerly known as The British Petroleum Company) and its partners. Among the key factors that contributed to the disaster were 'poor communications' and a failure 'to share important information.'

The reason for the dismissal of Piyasvasti Amranand from the post of CEO, Thai Air, in May 2012 remained wrapped in mystery for quite some time. But the media later quoted the airline's chairman as saying that 'communication problems between Piyasvasti and the board were hampering the company's effort to meet [its] profit target.'

Groysberg and Slind chose to view these lapses as 'case notes from the field of communication studies.' The two scholars wondered...'how many (business) leaders appreciate the risks that come with taking a lax approach to communication management—with failing to manage the way that ideas and information flow within their organizatin'?

Reluctance to change and communicate openly and effectively is the perfect recipe for business failure. Unfortunately, Nepal's old-style business is deeply affected by this malaise. It's time we changed and opened up.

Nepal's Women Entrepreneurs

May 2016

Mala Thapa Magar had a tough life. Her parents separated when she was just three months old. Today, barely out of her teens, she heads Himalayan Allo Udhyog at Budhanikantha which is worth Rs. 3 million and provides employment to around two dozen persons. Working on a leased 763-square-metre plot, she managed to accomplish this in four years.

Mala started the enterprise of natural fabric production in a partnership in 2009 but struck out on her own in 2012 with a one lakh investment. She procures natural fibres like allo and hemp from farmers in Sindhupalchok, Bajura, Bahjang and Dang and converts them into fabric which now has buyers in Nepal and abroad. Educated in the school of hard knocks, Mala was quick to foresee the growth in the natural fabric market. She withstood the ups and downs of business with the conviction that problems arise only to be solved. A true entrepreneur should have grit and gumption. Mala had those in abundance.

Lesson: Entrepreneurs are quick to identify opportunities and use them despite formidable challenges. Baby steps one day turn into giant strides.

Rekha Sunaur chose to go against conventional wisdom and even suffer threats of divorce from her Gulf-based husband who was dead opposed to her plan for the Dhaka weaving business. The male-dominated Nepali society makes it difficult for enterprising women to follow their dreams. But Rekha, an SLC pass-out, pursued her vision.[1] She had debts to clear. She had no customer relationship skills. In fact, she did not know how to talk to customers when she attended her first exhibition in Kathmandu; all her shawls remained unsold. But Rekha did not give up her dream to be her own master. She received training in all aspects of the weaving business from production to marketing and started with a measly amount of Rs. 3500 at Sindhupalchok. Her unit now produces not just shawls but also saris, scarves, mufflers and caps. She employs 10 persons today, saves close to Rs. 20,000 every month and plans to share her expertise by launching a network of Dhaka weaving centres. The same *pati parmeshwar* now wants to invest in her business!

Lesson: Entrepreneurs follow their heart with passion and refuse to be daunted by challenges. They continuously upgrade their skills to remain competitive. Having helped themselves, they believe in helping others.

Victims of the civil war, Rama Lamichane from Sindhupalchok and Krishna Basnet from Solukhumbu are running their mushroom farming business together with fair success in Kapan. They had just enough money to plough in Rs. 2 lakh into the project. They reaped Rs. 3 lakh at the end of the season.

But a mushroom farmer's life is tough. They have to get up at 3 a.m. to supply the produce to the wholesale market by 4.30 a.m. day after day. Initially, they used to carry their daily produce on a push-cart which was later replaced by a common scooty.

---

[1]SLC or the School Leaving Certificate refers to a national-level examination that all tenth graders in Nepal take before they graduate to the last two years of high school.

Mushroom farming is a risky affair; the produce can get easily damaged or destroyed. Maintaining a uniform production cycle requires tremendous care and labour. But Rani and Krishna do most of the work themselves and employ just four workers in a year. They believe that only prudent risk taking can ensure profits and growth. It is better to be an entrepreneur than an employee, proclaim the duo.

Lesson: Entrepreneurs know that gain demands pain. Therefore, starting one's own business is not for the faint-hearted. No work related to the enterprise is below one's dignity, including pushing a cart.

Lalita and Chandra Prasad Pandey both received a bachelor's degree in agriculture. Love for progressive and commercial farming led to marriage in 2013. They started with hybrid tomato seeds on just 685 square feet at village Kottimal in district Kavrepalanchowk. The place is about three hours from Kathmandu. Trained in agricultural science as they are, they planted the seeds under two plastic tunnels costing Rs. 30,000 each. The result was there to see in six months. The couple's efforts fetched them Rs. 340,000. Lalita plays an active role in the entire cultivation process. The neighbours, who used to be openly sceptical of modern agricultural techniques, are now keen on following the Pandey pattern. Chandra and Lalita are happy agriculture is no longer looked down upon as a profession in their region. In fact, it has earned a new respect.

Lesson: Entrepreneurship is all about thinking out of the box and being innovative. Tested modern ways of production enhance productivity and set the foundation for bigger enterprises.

Women who have the entrepreneurial fire burning in them must have already heard of Laxmi Sharma, who was Nepal's first woman auto-rickshaw driver, and went on to set up the country's first button factory, Laxmi Wood Craft Udhyog, in 1982. Kunjana Mishra of Kunj Artistic Beads and fashion designer Subhexya Bhadel, whose dresses have adorned several beauty pageant winners and whose signature garment line is making a mark, are also known pioneers in women entrepreneurship. Subhexya was dissuaded from entering fashion designing as her near and dear ones saw no 'scope' in it unlike established and conventional careers in medicine, engineering, teaching, government service, etc. She slogged, at times scrounging for funds to buy even thread and needles, and proved the world wrong.

Lesson: Entrepreneurs are strong personalities with full faith in the path they have chosen. They may fail, but they make every failure a stepping stone to success. They defy decaying social norms and business practices and chart their own course.

I could go on and on. But I wonder why I need to do so. Almost the entire informal sector, which is a major chunk of any economy, more so in Nepal, is run by private entrepreneurs. And I am not talking of big business companies and groups. I am talking of the grocery shops, fruit sellers, eateries, coaching centres, gyms, etc. which dot our markets and pavements in cities, towns and villages.

Have we noticed that a high percentage of such outlets are run by women, thanks to the migration of a large number of our young males to the Gulf and other countries? No doubt, the latter do remit money to Nepal. But many economic experts are of the view that the slow growth of our economy and virtually negative growth of the farm sector is because most able-bodied men are abroad. On top of that, most Nepali migrants are largely among those who provide unskilled and semi-skilled services abroad, the economic returns for which do not match the loss of their physical presence and consequent contribution to the country.

Nepal's economy is mostly being run by women. We need to rid them of social and regulatory shackles to let a million entrepreneurial women thrive and revive the country.

The Confucius Way To Grand Success

July 2016

Time is a great healer. The nightmarish memories of the April 2015 temblor are gradually fading. But one look at the remnants of the heart-rending devastation and horror descends again.

The political instability, which has only increased after the formulation of the Constitution in the wake of the quake, is adding to public ire and misery. The deeply divided government and a fractured political class have yet to choose between rehabilitation and reconstruction.

Meanwhile, worthwhile relief work remains stalled. The nation is clueless about the government's blueprint for meeting this daunting challenge. International donors seem more than perplexed at the delays and virtual paralysis in execution. How long will friendly countries and other donor organizations stand by their pledges when our officialdom itself refuses to stir out of somnolence?

What is wrong with us? If even a catastrophe of this scale and political turmoil cannot galvanize the state and also, to a great extent, citizens into purposeful, meaningful and concerted action, then what will? Work that should have begun yesterday is still nowhere on the horizon. Even concrete plans remain a mystery. That apart, we know very well that even the best of plans remain just that without the will and capability to execute them.

Are we culturally handicapped to handle crises in right earnest?

When I talk of culture I am implying a mindset which makes a nation goal-oriented, productive and progressive—the basic requirement for turning into a developed or advanced country. Work culture, in a nutshell.

Students of economics are well aware of the role of Protestantism in the emergence of capitalism, currently the world's most popular economic doctrine, in sixteenth-century Europe. German sociologist, economist and politician Max Weber demonstrated this effectively in his most influential work *The Protestant Work Ethic and the Spirit of Capitalism* in 1905.

Close to home, various adaptations of the teachings of Chinese philosopher Confucius (551–478 BC) have shaped the economic ideology, work ethics and destiny of countries like China, Japan, South Korea, Singapore, etc. Languishing as virtual subsistence economies towards the end of the 1940s, these countries are the real Asian tigers now. They are at the top of the heap having registered astounding economic growth, infrastructure development and social progress. What is common to these trailblazers? A past of either deprivation or devastation, and adherence to indigenously customized teachings of the Great Master Confucius. Defying formidable odds, these countries have created and followed enviable work cultures. Their systems are by no stretch of the imagination flawless but they have managed to give their citizens a life many countries, Nepal included, merely dream of.

Charlie Caruso,[2] who has researched the stupendous rise of the Chinese economy since 1980, found five traits which have become

---

[2]Charlie Caruso, the founder and CEO of PuggleFM, an online radio and podcasting station for parents and families.

integral to Chinese work culture, thanks to Confucius' profound influence.

According to Caruso, 'Crisis in the Chinese language literally translates to a combination of danger and opportunity. Every "crisis" poses a potential opportunity to the Chinese, only if that "danger" is managed properly.' The Chinese think positively and are always ready to embrace change. They also remain prepared to face the worst because, as Confucius observed, 'Success depends upon previous preparation and without preparation there is sure to be failure.'

Strategy is most vital to the Chinese way of business and life. Even the smallest business move is rooted in one's business strategy. 'If you think in terms of a year, plant a seed; if in terms of ten years, plant trees; if in terms of 100 years, teach the people,' said Confucius. Another gem from the Great Master: 'Without feelings of respect, what is there to distinguish men from beasts?' That is why Japanese and Korean societies are highly collectivistic. Filial piety prevails. Group orientation and team spirit are predominant. No wonder a company head treats employees as family members and terms like 'the Toyota family', 'the Hyundai family' or 'the Samsung family' sound true.

Korean and Japanese children are taught to act in harmony with the surrounding order. Therefore, working together on a universal, rather than an individual basis becomes second nature as they grow up. Group orientation and loyalty to the group is nurtured, giving the individual a social identity and a feeling of security. The rewards of service also go to the group. Therefore, team spirit flourishes and the most formidable of business projects and social objectives are accomplished.

In line with Confucian principles, Korean and Japanese behemoths offer their employees total integration within their structures. Take for example, the Toyota Technological Institute—an institute created by Japanese automotive major Toyota for its workers and even outsiders with some industrial knowledge and experience. Korean *chaebols* (major business conglomerates) indoctrinate new employees to consider their workplaces as a family.

Confucian principles, which have undergone change and indigenization in the recent past, were very much at play when Japan and Korea managed to recover rather quickly from the repeated financial crises which rocked the world in the late 2000s. Political and business elites collaborated and mobilized society to combat the challenges head-on. Singapore, with its largely Chinese-origin leadership, has much to thank Confucius for vis-à-vis its tremendous economic success and social accomplishments despite its tiny size. Vietnam too is following the Great Master's footsteps and tasting success despite the devastation it suffered in the long-drawn-out war with the US in the late 1960s and early 1970s.

Keen observers of these Asian economies understand well how Confucian values have permeated all spheres of life in these top-drive countries. At the same time, vices too are breaching the value system. But the core DNA will take time to get corroded.

On the other hand, what value system and work culture is Nepal following? Right now, the political class is deeply divided. Personal ambitions, it seems, will not allow the polity to settle down in the near future. Corruption remains unabated. Team spirit in factories remains a mirage. Strikes and *bandas* continue to dog industrialists, businessmen and the common folk. Yet all are crying hoarse proclaiming their commitment to nationalism and patriotism.

Nepal considers China a good friend. But we are not willing to listen to the Chinese Great Master who is revered across the world irrespective of nationality and racial heritage.

Is anybody listening?

Yoga Betters Your Business

August 2016

The International Day of Yoga was celebrated with great enthusiasm and hope in more than 150 countries around the globe on 21 June. From Times Square in New York to the Great Wall of China to science expedition centres in the Antarctica, millions practised yogic *asanas* and meditation techniques not just for personal well-being but for the overall welfare of today's stressed and strife-torn society.

Contrary to popular perception, yoga does much more than heal physical ailments and mental problems. The Sanskrit word 'yoga' means 'union'. But union with what? Yoga unites us with our inner being. It facilitates self-actualization or self-realization. It makes us better humans who are not easily rocked by the excesses of success and failure and who see 'self' in everybody else. The bonding this creates among all living beings is the real purpose of yoga and, certainly, the need of the day when religious bigotry, hate campaigns and terrorism are hogging headlines every day.

The United Nations Organization recognized the healing and uplifting attributes of the science of yoga and celebrated the first International Day of Yoga on 21 June 2015 with the support of

177 countries. And the tradition continues despite opposition from some religious extremists who refuse to acknowledge the scientific core of yoga. They demonize the ancient tradition as a means to propagate what they call Hinduism. However, their bluff has been called by medical doctors, biochemists, psychologists and other science experts from different countries, whose extensive research has established the scientific fundamentals of yoga. Today more and more people are embracing the practice of yoga, particularly in the advanced and relatively higher educated western world. No wonder, the International Day of Yoga 2016 turned out to be a unique secular celebration involving millions of human beings irrespective of nationality, religion, caste, creed and ideology. Indeed, yoga is becoming a way of life.

While the grand success of the 21 June celebrations was widely reported, what escaped the media's radar was the corporate world's active involvement in the event. In fact, the business world has been the most eager and active practitioner of yoga, and that too for years. The reason being that work-related stress has become an integral part of modern corporate life. Competition has intensified. Constant change has become a norm. Most business executives operate in an environment of ambiguity. The realm of certainty is history. And so is the physical, mental, emotional and spiritual well-being of the typical globalized manager. The higher he rises, the greater the challenges he faces. All this takes a toll on his physical and mental health. Personal burnouts occur all too often. Productivity suffers. Company bottom lines take a hit. Industries bear the brunt. The economy trundles downhill. All victims of stress, the silent killer!

And how it maims managers and businesses! Here are some statistics gleaned from US research reports on work-related stress.

(i) More than $300 billion a year are spent to take care of stress-linked ailments among corporate rank and file.

(ii) Close to 80 per cent office-goers regularly experience physical ailments. Absenteeism is rising.

(iii) Three-fourth of employees are battling with psychological issues. Anxiety, panic, depression, sleeplessness, mental breakdown, etc. are common. One-third complain of extreme stress. Decision-making gets impaired. Unhappy workers are 10 per cent less productive.

(iv) Almost 48 per cent employees feel stress has increased over the last five years. Constant pressure to achieve success is grievously impacting even the most robust of minds.

(v) Family bonds are taking a hit. Relationships are failing as business is taking precedence over personal commitments. Divorces are increasing. Children caught in this vicious cycle are getting traumatized for life. Generations are paying the price for corporate stress.

A recent report in *The Times of India* states, 'Employee meltdowns are haemorrhaging cash and India Inc. has realized it's cost effective to invest in health and wellness of the workforce.' The Society of Human Resource Management (SHRM) focused on the IT and ITeS, banking and finance, and travel and hospitality industries in India in the study which revealed that a banking/finance company, with an average employee base of 5,000 takes a hit of about INR 100 crore in productivity losses due to stressed manpower. 'For an IT/ITeS company, with an average employee base of 10,000, the loss is about Rs. 50 crore. And for a company with an average employee base of 2,000 operating in the travel and hospitality space, it's just over Rs. 10 crore. The productivity losses escalate as one moves to high stress sectors,' the report added.

Data from Indraprastha Apollo Hospitals, New Delhi, shows that almost 70 per cent business executives visiting its units are suffering from stress-related diseases, and the number is on the increase. Fortis

Healthcare, New Delhi, tells a similar tale. Renowned heart surgeon Dr Devi Shetty, who started Narayana Hrudayalaya Health City in Bangalore and the Rabindranath Tagore International Institute of Cardiac Sciences in Kolkata, says stress is tightening its grip on Indian corporate executives fast. Another leading cardiologist, Dr Naresh Trehan echoes the same sentiments. He himself practises breathing exercises in his car on his way to work. To combat the adverse impact of the fast-paced corporate life on their executives, Intel, Snapdeal, Jabong, Infosys, Maruti Suzuki and many other Indian companies have ardently taken to yoga.

Ms. Melissa Thompson, an independent producer for CNN who has been propagating the benefits of incorporating yoga in the corporate world, points out that many companies like Forbes, General Electric (GE), Apple, Google, Chase Manhattan Bank, Home Box Office (HBO), Nike, etc. have adopted the practice. Thompson asserts that yoga increases energy and reduces fatigue; alleviates physical ailments like aches or pains associated with traumatic brain injury, carpal tunnel, neck strain, shoulder stiffness, arthritis, etc.; relieves mental and emotional stress which accounts for 90 per cent of all visits to doctors and which, if left unaddressed, is known to lead to diabetes, cancer and heart conditions; improves concentration and focus, enabling managers to deal better with stressful deadlines, back-to-back and never ending meetings and the general corporate chaos; helps with creativity, thus facilitating out-of-the-box solutions; and increases productivity and enhances morale.

The Harvard Mental Health Letter too has documented many findings of the successful impact of yoga, especially Sudarshan Kriya, on anxiety, post-traumatic stress disorder and depression. A low-cost and effective recipe for happy and more productive managers, indeed!

Office Politics!

October 2016

That office politics plays havoc with corporate performance is too clichéd a comment to deserve repetition. But sometimes one needs to keep shouting from the rooftops to be heard. Even then there is no guarantee that it will really impact office politics addicts. So deep-rooted is this malpractice.

But who are the diehard practitioners of office politics? The incompetent and the undeserving, driven by unreasonable ambition and envy. Unable to make their mark on merit, they seek to rise up the corporate ladder through politicking in their departments, divisions and the organization. So good are they at this game that many times they succeed in their designs too. What a tragedy!

Decades of experience in running businesses in Nepal has brought me in touch with counterparts and partners in the subcontinent as well as in more advanced countries. I find office politics to be all-pervasive. It seems to be driven by the baser instincts among humans. However, it is not that intense where merit is the touchstone of success and where processes and systems inhibit individual discretion. The man on the top too plays a big role in keeping office politics in check.

Analysing this universal phenomenon in depth, I feel it is inevitable to some extent—while you cannot rule out office politics it can certainly be contained. After all, persons from diverse social and educational backgrounds work in an office or at a workplace. Their goals and interests too differ. Yet, organizational success lies in aligning individual goals with the organizational goals. Given what human nature is all about, this is easier said than done.

Ensuring that the organization's goals and the rank and file's interests remain on the same page requires a major change in corporate culture. An organization truly takes shape when all its stakeholders, particularly employees, realize the need to pursue a common goal. It is imperative that employees work in unison with full faith in the goals decided for the organization even though these may differ from time to time in keeping with the business environment. Therefore, there should be the willingness and flexibility to accept change and mould one's way of working. However, this happens only when the top leadership is able to convince employees that the organizational goals take full care of their interests too. This calls for a win-win orientation and transparency which, in turn, can ensure a positive ambience.

Let's come back to the prevalence and root causes of workplace politics. Why does office politics arise and then strike roots? Simply because undeserving employees resort to misusing their power to gain undue attention and popularity at the workplace. They perceive this as a means to move up the ladder little realizing that this does not help in the long run.

Merit ultimately prevails. But in the meanwhile well-meaning employees get hurt and feel compelled to seek jobs in better administered companies. The organization suffers. Attrition rises. Invariably, the competent ones are the first to flee. The rotten apples remain because they have no takers; they continue to swear by loyalty.

Replacing a good worker with a new one costs the organization dearly in more ways than one. The entire work cycle gets disrupted and takes time to return to normal. Persons with the required competencies are not easily available. Overall staff morale takes a hit. The top management is viewed as callous and apathetic to the genuine needs of efficient and competent employees. 'Yes-men/women seem to be the winners. Indeed, a very dangerous image for a company.

Typical masters at office politics show different behavioural patterns. Let me roughly categorize them:

1) *Limelight seekers:* They hate working hard. They resort to nasty politics by creating a negative image of their competitors specifically, and all co-workers, in general. The objective is to be in the good books of the bosses. Unfortunately, they often succeed especially when the bosses are immature, inefficient and feudal-minded. The feudal mindset is in evidence even in leading western companies. This is more individual-centric than culture-centric.

2) *Personal relationship exploiters:* Though it is quite difficult to keep personal bonds entirely out of the workplace, their undue interference in office can play havoc. People tend to favour their friends, relatives and neighbours. Intimate personal relationships in the workplace have often led to major scandals, big losses to the company because of the consequent lapses in commitment, and long-term damage to the company's reputation, which keeps potential competent employees from joining the organization.

3) *Trust in sceptics:* Trust between the employer and employees as well as among employees themselves is the bedrock of organizational efficiency and productivity. But because of an organization's inherent culture, often doubt, apprehension and scepticism emerge stronger than its positive aspects. Employees, mainly senior managers, choose to remain in their silos or shall I say ivory towers. The flow of vital workplace information gets disrupted. The right hand does not know what the left

hand is doing. Therefore coordination, which is the mantra of organizational success, becomes dysfunctional. The office politicking types exploit the situation to their advantage and manage to sow seeds of suspicion. A mature management team can salvage the situation by building a trusting organization. The bosses can do this by slashing hierarchy, making the company flatter or more horizontal, conducting open houses, creating secured digital channels of communication, and most importantly, letting go of their false egos.

4) *Naughty guys' tools:* Manipulation, bullying, pulling strings with the 'managed and massaged masters', blame game, gossip, backstabbing, leg pulling, stealing credit, demeaning others' achievements, etc. are freely put to use by seasoned office politics players. Very soon, friends turn foes. Team members stop helping each other. The team spirit goes for a toss and with it also the very concept of organization. Tension, conflicts and jealousy flourish. Uncalled for criticism and cribbing become the norm. The joy of work is lost and the smallest of daily assignments become drudgery. Negativity settles in and the company starts heading for decline and perhaps doom.

Hollywood movies like *Boiler Room, The Working Girl, Up in the Air, 9 to 5, Office Space, Smartest Guys in the Room* and *The Intern* have managed to capture workplace politics, warts and all. In fact, I feel these films are a must-see for working and aspiring corporate executives. But the million-dollar question is: how to keep office politics within permissible and tolerable limits, at least in our part of the world. It has to be admitted that the existing management style in Nepal is not much to crow about.

First and foremost, we need to understand and accept the importance of Human Resource Development (HRD) in Nepal's business and industry world. Alas, the prevailing mindset of business heads is not exactly amenable to this idea. They prefer to continue with their arbitrary and ad hoc style.

As such, Nepal is a resource-scarce country. It does not have either the means or the regulatory framework to import and install state-of-the-art technology in its factories. Besides, the size and scale of our manufacturing units is too small compared to the neighbouring countries. So that leaves us with just one resource to grow our businesses—human resource (HR).

But Nepal hardly has any truly qualified HR managers, let alone experts. Our HRD policies and systems are archaic and have little relevance to the changing business scenario around us. Containing office politics is a skill which most of our HR managers have yet to acquire. Instead the HR office, being whatever of a power centre it is, functions as the fountainhead of gossip. Confidentiality and trust-building do not figure prominently on HR teams' agendas. The cane-wielding headmaster continues to be their ideal.

Making things worse is the feudal approach of the top management. Yes-men are preferred over competent and qualified professionals. Strangely enough, even company promoters and owners tend to do this though they have no reason to feel insecure because of their hired managers. Elsewhere, business tycoons take pride in recruiting and retaining professionals smarter than themselves in specialized functions. This is the first step towards corporatization of business. But Nepali business seems to be afraid of taking this first baby step.

No wonder sycophants and hangers-on continue to occupy major positions and perpetuate office politics. Nepal needs a paradigm shift in the way it does business.

Whither Values For Business?

November 2016

Ideally, business and ethics should walk hand in hand. Unfortunately, they seldom do.

The last few decades have witnessed the simultaneous rise of big business and bigger scams. Ironically, the same period has seen the emergence of several industrial, business and technology icons who have changed the face of the earth. By creating large-scale employment, immense business opportunities for medium and small entrepreneurs, wealth for ordinary shareholders and bodies dedicated to corporate social responsibility, these so-called capitalists have done more for society than many self-proclaimed socialists and communists.

Yet business and profit continue to be dirty words in public perception and perceptions are powerful. Reinforced over a period of time, they become an integral part of collective memory which is not easy to alter, let alone erase and rewrite.

And when you live in Nepal, which figures so high on the world corruption index, it is easy to see corruption even where none exists. Don't we keep seeing ghosts when none exist?

But isn't it strange that while we are ever ready to discuss business ethics, we do not care much about ethics in politics? I am not trying to build a case for businessmen, good or bad. I simply wish to point out the fact that while there is no dearth of court and police cases against different sections of the business class in the country, cases against politicians are few and far between. Also, the ones which are launched rarely reach a logical conclusion. I will not stoop to elaborating on the name-and-shame game, and I need not because the licentiousness of the ruling class is an open secret in Nepal.

The reason why I am raising this issue in a business magazine is that the socio-economic root cause of corruption needs to be looked into comprehensively. Yes, there is corruption and violation of ethics in business in Nepal. But it is less, or may be, at par with any other social sections—certainly the country's ruling elite comprising politicians and administrators currently, and the monarchy in the past. Business is rooted in society and is ruled by the prevailing culture—political, bureaucratic, administrative, social and even historical.

Readers would appreciate that the country's business class, including industry owners, senior managers, executives and even small shopkeepers, needs to abide by a host of rules and regulations, which are most of the time unthought of, arbitrary and ad hoc. With lack of transparency pervading all our systems in Nepal, the powers that be at different levels have ample leeway for arm-twisting businessmen, traders, shopkeepers and the like. Greasing palms has turned into a fine art. If you don't, you run the risk of slipping into business oblivion. So for sheer survival, many from the business world have fallen in line with the systems promoted and propagated by the ruling elite. Experts at manipulating, manoeuvring and tending to itching palms have risen to great heights.

Truth be said, no business person, owner or employee likes being corrupt or unethical. But business folk have not descended from another planet. They are products of the prevailing socio-economic culture. Personal and professional lives overlap and impact each other. In the process, the two become one. Unethical practices become acceptable to the individual as he sees no great stigma attached to them. Corruption appears to be a way of collective life. The individual, in this context the business promoter and manager, sees the protectors of public morality steeped in corruption and going scot-free. He hardly finds any ideals to follow.

That my contention has substance is obvious from the high levels of honesty in social and business life in Scandinavian and Nordic countries like Sweden, Norway, Denmark, Finland, Iceland and the Netherlands, and their adherence to ethics and humanitarian principles. No wonder these countries are viewed as perfect playfields for existing and aspiring businessmen and managers. There is rule of law. There are no ethical dilemmas. That is the perfect environment for business. Lapses do happen. But those are exceptions and not the rule. Why? Because business ethics and principles gradually become part of the national psyche.

In Nepal, on the other hand, business ethics is not even a full-fledged course in MBA classes even today. We tell students about the beautiful flowers and fruits of the business garden. We talk only about rewards and enticements. We create unrealistic dreams for them. We goad them to achieve those senseless goals without caring for the means they would use in this mad pursuit. But we have hardly a word highlighting the roots of business—the ethics, principles, dedication, perseverance, innovation, lateral thinking et al. We offer mere skills, those too bookish, dated and outmoded. But what about the much-needed value system? The need for it does not even seem to occur to us.

Management researchers Donaldson and Werhane[3] (1993) have described ethics as 'a study of the human values of people in business

---

[3]Thomas Donaldson and Patricia Hogue Werhane, *Ethical Issues in Business: A Philosophical Approach*, Upper Saddle River, New Jersey, Prentice Hall, 1993.

practice! Several other experts like Kohlberg (1981[4] and 1987[5]), Borkowski and Ugras[6] (1992), Dees and Starr[7] (1992), and others have written that virtue is based on principles of justice which people imbibe over a lifetime and it becomes embodied in social institutions. That is why it has been surmised that ethics is the study of whatever is good for humans. In fact, Fatoki and Merembo[8] (2012) highlighted the vital need for a business organization to follow a code of business to ensure higher profitability and performance.

I recall that the World Forum for Ethics in Business Excellence had organized a conference in Kathmandu on 17 January 2014. The topic was 'Business Ethics for a Prosperous Nepal'. Over 600 delegates had participated. On 15 January, a talk and discussion was held on the role of women in instilling human values and ethics in society. It is obvious that management experts have higher trust in women when it comes to encouraging human values in society.

But what since then? Little that I am aware of despite being at the epicentre of business and commerce.

However, given the current environment not many may pay heed to the need for being ethical. Corruption fetches quick money. But countries which have really made it big in business are the ones that remained wedded to a pro-humanity value system. There is an age-old

[4]Lawrence Kohlberg, *Essays on Moral Development: Vol. 1*, The Philosophy of Moral Development, San Francisco, Harper and Row, 1981.

[5]Anne Colby et al., *The Measurement of Moral Judgment: Vol 1*, Theoretical Foundations and Research Validation, New York, Cambridge University Press, 1987.

[6]Susan Borkowski and Yusuf Ugras, *The Ethical Attitudes of Students as a Function of Age, Sex and Experience*, Journal of Business Ethics. 11. 961-979. 10.1007/BF00871962, 1992.

[7]J.G. Dees and J. A. Starr, *The Organization Makers: A Behavioral Study of Independent Entrepreneurs*, New York, Appleton-Century-Croft, 1992.

[8]O. Fatoki and M. Merembo, *An investigation into the attitudes toward business ethics by university students in South Africa*, African Journal of Business Management, 5865-5871, 2012.

saying: honesty is the best policy. It may sound jaded to some today. But old is still gold. It embodies the proven wisdom of mankind.

Management Education in a Mess

February 2017

Management education in our part of the world, specifically Nepal, is a far cry from what real business needs. No wonder both aspiring managers and potential employers find themselves on parallel tracks which never, or at best, rarely meet.

As a consequence, the nation's managerial productivity remains abysmally low. Compared to most other countries we cut a sorry figure. This also explains the abundant involvement of foreign consultants for most of our business and government projects.

Management education alone cannot be blamed for the present state of affairs. There is something basically rotten about our entire educational system, beginning from the primary level. However, this forum is appropriate only to dissect and discuss the innards of our business and management education institutions.

No Nepalese educational institution has ever figured in *The Times* (UK) Higher Education World University Ranking and the *Financial Times* (UK) Top 100 Business Schools. These are the world's most recognized and accepted rankings of educational institutions. In fact, none of our educational organizations finds a place in Asian or even subcontinental rankings. Though people are aware of the names of a couple of our older universities, our business schools continue to wallow in oblivion. Indeed a strange and heart-rending reality for the land where Gautam the Buddha was born, where Himalayan rishis and munis live, and the closest neighbour of the country to which the *Arthashastra* (classic treatise on economic policy and statecraft written by Kautilya, also known as Chanakya) belongs. For geopolitical reasons, Nepal has been cosying up to China, an ancient land of wisdom. But the masters of our educational policy and administration have yet to understand, interpret and imbibe the tenets of the Great Master Confucius. Truth be stated: we are confused.

While Nepal has displayed intemperate eagerness to receive financial aid, grants and largesse from our neighbours and others who are in a charitable mood, we have been apathetic towards importing their knowledge systems. Myopically focused on our daily needs, we have never cared to think of tapping the fountainheads of knowledge and education to create a brighter new generation and nation. We remain all too happy sending our unskilled and semi-skilled youth as the lowest-paid labour to distant lands where they get exploited as subhumans and often perish. In fact, their absence from our low population country has disrupted the social equilibrium as well.

But the powers that be remain happy as long as the remittances from our migrants contribute more than handsomely to our gross domestic product—30 per cent to be precise. How long will our fatigued and tormented youth continue to feed us with their sweat and toil? We are living on blood money. Let us accept the fact and equip ourselves for the new world's knowledge-driven economy. For that we need to overhaul our educational system, from the bottom up.

But I need to revert to the article's focus on Nepal's business and management education. The bane of the current system is its excessive or rather total dependence on bookish learning. If books alone could teach, then people could have become pilots and astronauts by relevant reading. Scientific innovation would have happened without toiling in laboratories. Life-altering economic theories would have emerged without extensive and intensive field studies lasting years and decades. Management tools and systems would have been ours without scholars spending years on industrial shop floors. Or, perhaps you could have learnt swimming without stepping into the water but by reading some book like 'Ten steps to great championship swimming'!

Being at the epicentre of industry, business and commerce, I know how difficult it is to get even a good stenographer, secretary, assistant, let alone a bright young manager. There is a gross mismatch between B-school teaching and the real requirements of business and industry. Why is this so? Alas, it is a big why.

For one, Nepal does not have the faculty to teach real business in classrooms. It is generally believed that teachers are, or should be, appointed on the basis of their academic excellence. However, that is not usually the case as we are a country where ties, relationships and extraneous interests in appointments override core factors. And even if academic excellence is the touchstone, this does not guarantee a good education that particularly in the field of business must keep up with the latest developments. Course toppers, who often achieve the feat by mugging notes and regurgitating the same in their answer sheets (as is the custom in our educational system), do not always make the best teachers. Teaching is an art which, may I say, is a natural talent.

Two, a true academician is an indefatigable seeker of knowledge. He revels in backbreaking study and research and adds to the existing repository of knowledge. No wonder the western world picks up the best minds from across the globe, provides them the best facilities and environment and creates new knowledge in diverse academic spheres, both pure and applied. That leads to new patents, sponsorship by business and industry, and subsequent growth and prosperity for society and the nation.

Research in Nepal is largely a cut-and-paste affair, thanks to the World Wide Web. It has scant practical utility. With a little scrutiny and monitoring, these scraps of paper and a little string pulling (a national pastime) can land one a university teaching job, which can last for three decades.

Even bright and dedicated scholars with a genuine love and ability for teaching get little exposure to the hurly-burly of real business and management. Only a few have participated in any significant business activity. Unlike other countries, I have yet to come across any teaching faculty in Nepal whom the business community would like to engage as consultant. Bookish knowledge, and that too half-baked, does not inspire any confidence among employers. Our B-school students, therefore, emerge out of their classes like the blind led by the blind.

This unfortunate situation could have been and can still be remedied to some extent if our management institutes try to expand and intensify their interaction with business houses or even government departments which are involved in social businesses and development activities. Real life case studies are conspicuous by their absence. Elsewhere, they form the basic tool of instruction. The near absence of the stress on entrepreneurship in curricula produces seekers of safe and cushy jobs whereas Nepal today needs job and wealth creators.

Start-ups are the flavour of today's business the world over, but our B-schools only train students for safe desk jobs. The world's top billionaires today have toiled, repeatedly fumbling and rising again in dingy rooms and garages till just a few decades ago. And this glorious tradition is continuing. However, thanks to IT-enabled technology, the start-up trend is spreading like wildfire in the developing world. Our B-schools need to produce venturesome pupils. Established business conglomerates are today looking out for management students who are imbued with the 'intrapreneurial' spirit—the fire and the ability to lead and run departments or units within the conglomerate or company with a sense of ownership, driven by innovation and ethical governance. Such managers are known to have created miracles and changed the face of business houses.

Now the last but not the least important point: who will create these miraculous management institutes in Nepal? One may be prompted to come up with names of known academicians and scholars. But nothing could be further from reality. It is a known fact that our academic institutions are among the worst administered. Most of them are financial disasters and survive on government doles. In turn, the heads of these institutions are at the beck and call of their political and bureaucratic masters.

Nepal's management education needs visionary institution builders who are also equipped with proven administrative and managerial ability. Institution building and academic leadership is notches above writing research papers, lecturing students, creating timetables, organizing seminars, conducting convocations and the like.

The world has found that the functional heads of leading universities are not always professors. Nepal needs practitioners. They profess less and practise more.

Communicate or Perish!

March 2017

The popular perception about business is that it is simply the right mix of money, men and machines. All these are tangible entities which can be seen, felt and quantified. Money can help you with capital expenditure, that is, in setting up factories or service organizations, building employee-friendly offices and customer-centric systems and outlets, branding and promoting what you wish to make and sell. Appropriate manpower can ensure that your resources are optimally utilized for the growth of the organization, delivery of best possible products or services to different customer segments. Machines, today, pertain more to technology which has become the main driver of growth even in poor and developing countries which would rather promote employment than technology. But the business scenario today is such that one cannot do without technology. It has become an integral extension of our life. We cannot imagine our lives today without information technology and IT-enabled services like telecommunication, whether it be in Kathmandu, the higher reaches of the Himalayas, or the vast plains of the Terai belt.

Not just for business, technology is vital for mere sustenance and propagation of social welfare programmes. Contrary to popular perception of a few decades ago when technology was viewed as a job killer, it is now being accepted as an employment creator and enhancer.

But are the 3Ms—money, men and machines—enough to make a business enterprise succeed?

Rarely so!

Why?

Because men are not machines. They cannot be run with diesel, petrol, electricity and new means of alternative and renewable energy. Made of flesh and blood, humans give their best only when their hearts and minds are in the best shape and when their spirits are soaring. This is easier said than done. In fact, managing finance and technology is often easier than managing men. And who marshals money and machines? Manpower, or what has come to be known in modern management parlance as human resource or HR.

So what are Nepal's businesses doing to enhance their HR and, in the process, optimize their other resources like finance and whatever level of technology they are using? It may sound strange but it is true that the country's small and medium enterprises (SMEs) have displayed better skills and ability at managing their relatively small employee bases. One may argue that unlike established corporates and big business houses, SMEs are not bound by a plethora of rules and regulations. They are not bound to pay high salaries and allowances. But that, I feel, is not the real reason behind the HR-friendly behaviour visible in most Nepali SMEs which have created large-scale employment in the country's informal sector. The reason lies elsewhere. It now figures on the top of the latest global management literature. It is all about communication. The world follows the principles of communication religiously to build inter and intra-business bonds. Through structured and informal modes of communication, ultra-large, big and medium business enterprises seek to ensure that their HR remains on the same page, particularly about the most vital objectives, changing state of business, new challenges, required changes, etc.

Continuous corporate communication inspires employees to sincerely relate to the vision and mission of the organization. Otherwise, routine vision and mission statements remain mere high-sounding words to most workers. and staff. But once employees find themselves being kept abreast of the latest developments, good or challenging, in the company and the related markets, they start viewing themselves as stakeholders in the company. They start contributing their best to resolve emerging crises and face new market challenges. A person working on the shop floor for decades can often come up with technical solutions which would never strike the young or middle managers holding fancy qualifications. There is no substitute for experience.

Internal communication happens spontaneously in SMEs. Down from the proprietor to the load-heaving worker everyone has a good understanding of the state of the business and the market. Most SMEs are closely knit units, generally driven by a burning ambition to grow. They are, therefore, the most innovative too. Not chained by company hierarchy, rules, regulations, forms and documents, SMEs can afford to be nimble-footed. They can make changes much faster than files move in business conglomerates or government departments. No wonder SMEs are the largest employers the world over. Their role is unparalleled in Nepal where millions of our able-bodied youth migrate to India and distant lands to make a living and ensure two square meals for their families back home via remittances. In the process, the social fabric gets disrupted and it falls upon our womenfolk to run the family.

Go to any small or big market, bazaar or haat in Nepal and you will find mostly women running the show. And how well they do it despite occupying the lowest status in Nepalese society! While all that needs to be done to guarantee women their rightful place in society, may I say hardship and discrimination has imbued in Nepalese SME owners and entrepreneurs the grit and determination to carve out a niche for themselves. Devoid of any false notions of business hierarchy, office-linked arrogance and snobbery, Nepalese women are fast establishing themselves as masters of the common man's markets. Many of them have managed to scale up their businesses and entered into hitherto male-dominated domains like publishing, manufacturing, medical care, trading, banking, etc.

Women are natural communicators. They open their hearts, listen to others, share happiness and sorrow. Empathy comes naturally to them. They bring people together and invariably turn out to be better employers and co-workers.

Compared to them, I find male managers in Nepal to be highly hierarchy conscious. Like tigers protecting their territories, the typical Nepalese male manager prefers to remain in his silo, shooting orders through the phone and internet and once in a while in person. Bossing around is his passion. It is not for him to mingle with employees and co-managers, understand their needs and problems, acquaint them of the challenges being faced by the organization, and all else that could make things more open and transparent. Knowledge and information are power for him and he does not share them at any cost. The result is that corporates are riven with groups and coteries working at cross purposes. They are often so big that the right hand does not know what the left hand is doing. Also being multi-layered and huge they can afford to suffer and still sustain themselves despite such weaknesses. SMEs do not enjoy this luxury.

So the heavens fall in big business houses only when lack of communication causes major bottlenecks like cash flow issues, material supply disruption leading to production delay or stoppages, compliance issue violations prompting regulatory authorities to go for the company's jugular, etc. It's often too late by then.

What will the best of money, men and machines do when companies excel at keeping their mouths shut? The 3Ms have become a common denominator in the current scenario. Almost all big companies and business segments have access to these means and resources. I do not wish to name names, but we have seen multi-billion business transnationals in the neighbourhood and also in the advanced West come to grief because of sealed lips, lack of transparency and declining corporate governance. At the core of all such disasters has been misplaced, displaced or lost communication.

We don't have to go far to learn new lessons. Nepalese women running SMEs around us can be our best teachers. But will our male managers be able to swallow their egos and learn from the ladies?

The Hunt For the Cosy

May 2017

The craze for cushy government and corporate jobs is on the rise among our educated youth. Those straight out of colleges or B-schools aspire to para-drop into cosy cabins 'strategizing' for companies, little knowing that they are not even conversant with the day-to-day tactics of business. This mindset is typical of the subcontinent and some neighbouring regions where social status is determined more by the office you occupy than the actual work you do. This is most unfortunate and detrimental to the overall growth of the economy and business. The deleterious mentality needs to undergo change rapidly.

As an entrepreneur and industrialist with interests in diverse business domains, I constantly find myself besieged with requests and recommendations by parents, many of them very highly placed, for desk jobs for their children. The elders seem to be extremely concerned about keeping their tender children away from the sweat and grime of real business. Little do they realize that they are harming their progeny in the process. By keeping their fresh-out-of-college kids away from the hurly-burly of real business they are depriving the young ones of real education and training. Educational institutions can offer bookish knowledge but it needs to be practised on the shop floor, in markets and bazaars with dealers and distributors in far and remote towns and villages, through direct door-to-door selling, by conducting market surveys in the hinterland, by realizing company dues from reluctant stakeholders, by acting tough and smooth as well as smiling to maintain and nurture business ties...

Business is a school of hard knocks. And this schooling begins after students pass out with degrees and diplomas in management and other related disciplines. This is where the real business schooling begins. Those who excel here go on to earn name and pride sooner than later. Those bagging easy desk jobs through recommendations remain stuck there or soon find themselves unfit to meet real life business challenges. The cocooned cabin life comes to a sudden end. They quit or are asked to do so. They are compelled to start their professional lives afresh though much precious time has been lost by then. They find themselves lagging behind in their careers thereafter. Why do the children, and more importantly their resourceful parents, not realize the folly of overprotection?

I don't find this happening in the West. Of late, even our neighbouring countries have shown the trend of young people going in for a master's in management after considerable work experience. Several leading business schools do not even consider inexperienced college graduates. Unlike Nepal, management curriculum and pedagogy, that is, teaching methodology, is experience based abroad. Real and current business studies form the crux of professorial inputs and pupil participation.

How will a student understand production management if he has not spent time on the factory's shop floor and has never seen an assembly line at work? Can a person learn the intricacies of consumer behaviour without having interacted with customers herself? Can books alone inculcate a problem-solving attitude and ability if you are not used to tackling small and big business challenges before entering a management institute to further sharpen your skills with the latest research-based knowledge? Can HRD treatises generate in you empathy for company employees, develop an insight into organizational behaviour and equip you for handling sudden industrial unrest? In a nutshell, books cannot substitute experience gained from the ups and downs of corporate life. I, therefore, always advise students to experience business realities in factories, markets, business negotiations, government and regulatory offices before aspiring for managerial jobs in the corporate office. Frankly, bereft of such experience they will find themselves of no use at the corporate level. One who has not been in the battlefield cannot make a general.

The IIMs in India conduct the toughest test in the world for admitting students. Most of them are engineers from prestigious IITs and other leading institutions who pay fees from their savings or take education loans. Leading industrial behemoths, including MNCs, strive hard to recruit these bright students a semester before they pass out. Most of these students go on to become CEOs of top companies in their country and abroad.

But few studying management in Nepal would be aware that these students are made to undergo the most rigorous training in the smallest of towns and villages during their management traineeship and even after that. These bright stars from IIMs drawing multi-lakh and even crore-plus remuneration packages travel alongside tiny vans and even manual rickshaws with their company products to small *kirana* (small grocery) shops and stores in suburbs and villages. They spend time with shop owners sipping syrupy tea in dirty cups and *kullhars* (earthen cups) amidst a swarm of flies and dust and seek shelf space for their FMCG (fast-moving consumer goods) and industrial products or pharmaceuticals. This is real relationship management in action. This is real education. This is the mantra to success. Corporate assignments at the headquarters or regional office do not even figure in the initial career plans of these rising management stars. They know their time will come when they complete their *tapasya* (penance). It has been rightly said, 'First deserve then desire'. Unfortunately, few seem to pay heed to this age-old maxim in Nepal.

Today's youth also ignore another vital fact. Though all of them want to be ensconced in the air-conditioned confines of a corporate office, few remember that almost all mighty business houses and conglomerates have been built by entrepreneurs single-handedly. In Nepal, these great men toiled for years under the most tough and unfavourable circumstances and regimes to create new businesses which blossomed into business groups and conglomerates. Nepal's top businesses are a testimony and tribute to the pioneering spirit of this venerable tribe of gentlemen. My late father Lunkarandas ji was the one to set up the foundation of Nepal's largest multi-national business group. I have myself witnessed the hostile challenges which he had to encounter to carve out a place for the family business and then professionalize it. The risks he took in his venture then would drive the wits out of a professional business executive today.

While there is no denying the fact that entrepreneurs and only entrepreneurs have built the world economy, created wealth and employment and shared it with public holders of company shares and securities, very few youngsters in Nepal think of launching their own enterprises. They prefer the security of government service where there is little accountability. The next choice is a desk job in a reputed private entity. Our youth are not even remotely venturesome. When you avoid pain then you miss out on gain.

Ironically, the idols of the youth remain the likes of Bill Gates, Mark Zuckerberg, Steve Jobs, Dhirubhai Ambani, N.R. Narayana Murthy, and a host of entrepreneurs who have changed the face of the world. All of them had very humble beginnings. Even modern companies prefer entrepreneurial executives; they have come to be known as 'intrapreneur'. GE's former CEO Jack Welch figures at the top of this category.

And the informal sector in Nepal is run largely by lowly educated but gutsy women. They run tiny shops and stores, earn for their families and create jobs without investing big amounts. When will our educated youth draw inspiration from these ladies, show some daring and enter the business domain, fully prepared to conquer its vagaries and taste success? When will the global start-up revolution ignite their minds and hearts?

Nepal's educated youth needs to come out of their comfort zone before their passion and spirit totally evaporate and the country turns into a virtually fossilized entity.

Gyan on a Platter

June 2017

Most young managers seek to discover the mantra of success and shoot up the corporate ladder often faster than they deserve. Human desire and ambition know no bounds. Unfortunately, the secret to success is not available at discount bazaars and mega sales. But if you have the basic mettle and are willing to learn from self-made captains of business and industry, then the road to success can become smoother. However, listening to sane advice and abiding by it is easier said than done.

Going through a past issue of *Harvard Business Review (HBR)*, I happened to come across an insightful interview of Nagavara Ramarao Narayana Murthy who co-founded India's highly respected information technology multinational Infosys. Though an M.Tech from IIT Kanpur, Murthy launched Infosys with some of his colleagues from Patni Computers and friends virtually from scratch in 1981. They invested INR 10,000 to start the company and even that amount came from Murthy's wife Sudha.

Murthy took Infosys to great heights. It is India's sixth largest publicly traded company today. Murthy, 71, is now its Chairman

Emeritus with a net worth of $1.8 billion as per a 2015 assessment. By launching the employee stock option plan (ESOP) he ensured that even his driver could become a multi-millionaire. Yet he continued to lead a very simple life. Murthy is a significant philanthropist. Little wonder that *Fortune* magazine listed him amongst the 12 greatest entrepreneurs of our time. *Time* magazine described him as the father of the Indian IT sector. National and international honours have been conferred upon him by the dozen. Governments around the world seek his advice. So when N.R. Narayana Murthy speaks, the world listens. I wish to discuss this great man's views on leadership and management with young professionals.

At a time when the world, especially the youth, seems hypnotized by consumerism and hankers to acquire more and more, Murthy remains a staunch believer in a frugal and inexpensive lifestyle. He recounted to *HBR* what his father had told him very early in life: 'He (father) said if you cultivate inexpensive habits, you will not become a victim of money in later years. And, you will not fall into the trap of greed which leads you to do things that you will later regret.' Murthy never forgot what his father told him. As Infosys grew, he shared the company's wealth with employees through ESOPs and with lakhs of Infosys shareholders. He also always remembered his father's advice to read, which he did by borrowing books from the town library, and to listen to music, which he did by going to the municipal park where music was played on the public address system in the evening. All this came free for Murthy and his seven siblings who could not afford even these basic amenities during their childhood. Books, magazines and newspapers offered knowledge while music nourished sensitivity for the fine arts and aesthetics, all so essential to make a person complete. Another gem of advice from his father: 'Cultivate good friends and discuss interesting and useful things with these friends. These conversations do not cost you any money.'

And how handsomely did this wisdom pay back Murthy and

friends! They founded Infosys together and remained a team, with one friend taking over the helm from another who stepped down on reaching the age of retirement. No other company in the world can claim to have had such a smooth succession system. No wonder Infosys did not witness any fight for succession till all the original set of founders had retired.

In the course of the interview, Murthy brings to our notice an important lesson that he learnt from Professor J.G. Krishnayya (JGK), his boss at the Indian Institute of Management, Ahmedabad. 'He taught us the importance of starting every transaction on a zero base and not carrying the hysteresis of bias from prior transactions. Let me give you an example. From time to time, JGK and I would have a discussion on a technical issue. In the heat of excitement, we would say things that would not be appropriate. I was guilty of it more often than JGK. I would spend the night worrying that JGK had gotten upset with me. But the next morning when I met him, he would be smiling, affectionate and full of charm. He would behave as if that offending transaction did not happen. In fact, my colleagues at Infosys have observed me behaving exactly like JGK did. They know that my comments were purely on that issue and have nothing to do with the person involved,' Murthy told the *HBR* interviewer.

I find this sage-like suggestion from Murthy highly valuable in the Nepali context where we are known to nurse grudges on trivial issues. This is not confined to the business world alone. The malaise has affected our entire system, particularly the legislature, the executive and the judiciary. They are at loggerheads with one another most of the time over clash of egos and vested interests. The nation suffers. There seems to be no space for genuine differences of opinion and for gentlemanly discourse. To be honest, I see the same happening in the corporate world which is expected to be result oriented for sheer survival and growth. But in our feudal set-up, I often come across the best minds in business languishing by the side because they dared to challenge the viewpoint of their owner or superiors. Yes-men flourish while the business flounders.

In such circumstances, valid theses, arguments and data become irrelevant. In contrast to our pathetic state, Murthy always stuck to JGK's following advice, 'Young man, if you use data and facts to arrive at conclusions, then you will not be biased, you will not be opinionated, and you will be fair to the other person.' The advice, worth its weight in gold, was offered to Murthy by the wise professor way back in the late 1960s. And he practised it all his life. Murthy still tells youngsters, 'In God we trust. Everybody else brings data to the table.'

Following Donald Trump's ascendancy to the US presidency, these are not the best times for India's IT industry. Yet the market capitalization of Infosys stood at $36.6 billion on 31 March 2017. Such is the outcome of a hard data-based empirical approach to business. In Nepal, on the contrary, real figures and data largely remain a mystery wrapped in an enigma. Murthy's unflinching faith in data is rooted in the following gyan (wisdom) which he shares with all young professionals: '... I tell them... to practise honesty, integrity, decency and fairness. I communicate these values to them by the adage, "The softest pillow is a clear conscience". And, they understand that I am advising them to be honest, to be fair to others, to use data and facts, and not be biased.' This leads to transparency. Murthy stated, 'I use the adage, 'When in doubt, disclose' to communicate this powerful attribute of a value system. Transparency is a prime value attribute in the corporate world because good corporate governance depends on transparency. Transparency is also the hallmark of a good professional, a good human being and good citizen of any society.' Murthy also advises youngsters to equip themselves for operating in multi-cultural environments. The globalized world expects this attribute in all business managers. A multi-cultural mindset is the need of the hour.

Though appreciative of Indian managers' ability to work hard, Murthy expects more from them. He observed, '... Indian managers have to learn better the ability to move from being reactive problem solvers to proactive problem definers, or proactive solution definers. Indians are very hard working. They are reasonably smart. But by and large, Indian professionals expect their bosses to tell them in detail what needs to be done.'

How I wish that business managers in Nepal too would pay heed to Murthy's advice. They are far too prone to decisions and solutions being offered to them by either the promoters or the top management. This attitude only blunts and rusts their own ability and mental acumen. This is enough gyan from a living legend. Let our managers follow in Murthy's footsteps.

Looking For Successful Managers?

July 2017

Today's youth has fallen in love with instant gratification. They are addicted to two-minute noodles even when they have the option of savouring the ubiquitous noodle elaborately cooked in a myriad flavours and tastes. But the young seem to be in a tearing hurry especially when it comes to climbing the success ladder.

I find nothing wrong with this aspirational race but at times I wonder at the shortcuts young managers take to rise rapidly. I am saddened when I find many of these high climbers falling flat fast and hard. In the mad rush to get to higher designations they forget that with every high designation comes higher responsibility which demands solid experience, maturity, knowledge and skill sets. How will you have all this when you have been busy hopping from one post to the next higher one, caring little to learn on the way?

What happens if you go for a 100-metre dash without a warm-up? If you are lucky you develop just cramps. Otherwise you end up damaging a ligament or tendon banishing you from racing for months. Only the supremely stupid will try the Everest ascent without undergoing the customary acclimatization at the base camps. Career planning and growth in business management are no different.

A leading mentor to young business managers in the US was rather shocked when told by some of her mentees that companies should increase layers of management to ensure frequent promotions. The suggestion was not just ludicrous but also self-serving given the fact that the corporate world is fast moving towards flatter organizations, and hierarchical structures are being slashed.

The reigning wisdom is that managers should be known and recognized by their work content and job profile rather than by mere designations. On a more philosophical level, managers should derive greater satisfaction from the value they are adding to the organization and to their personal selves than from a high-sounding job title.

India's largest automobile maker, Tata Motors Ltd, has from this April reduced its 16-level hierarchy to a flat 5-level structure. Similar exercises have been in progress in Tata Steel's European operations and its behemoth IT unit Tata Consultancy Services (TCS).

Delayering is a worldwide trend and is not restricted to our region. In fact, it has been far more aggressive outside the subcontinent. Even a totalitarian country like China, which is also the world's largest growing economy, has recognized the benefits of making its companies adopt leaner and flatter management and employee structures.

Not too long ago, there was a proliferation of vice-presidents in western, mainly US, businesses. This was evident all the more in IT companies. IT and ITeS companies in the Indian subcontinent too copied their western counterparts till there came a time when people started joking that very soon there would be VPs for toilets, office décor and coffee stations as well. The designation lost its dignity and gravity. This happened because employee attrition levels used to be very high in the IT industry. Fancy designations were doled out to managers and IT experts to keep them within the fold. There was little correlation between a manager's designation and his actual role in the organization. However, the more stable and down-to-earth manufacturing sector did not fall prey to this pernicious trend. No wonder managerial designations there continue to command respect. The posts clearly signified the actual role, knowledge, experience and position of the person in the company. VPs were few and far between in the biggest of manufacturing companies. It is still so.

Are designations or 'external signposts' a real measure of success? Isn't the mad race for acquisition of these external marks a sign of insecurity and the unwillingness to learn and grow on the job? While only an in-depth socio-psycho-anthropological research may offer a plausible explanation of this conundrum, I can certainly share with young managers the pitfalls that bedevil the rat race for success (read 'flashy designations'). I have come across many young managers in a perpetual state of hurry. Some of them were fairly bright too. But their vaulting ambition knew no bounds. They wanted to climb ranks virtually every six months. Left to themselves, they would have ardently longed to become CEOs of major companies within six to seven years. They are the ones who get lured by run-of-the-mill or upstart outfits the fastest. The glitter and pull of the fancy post is overwhelming. Once tempted and trapped by such outfits, these so-called CEOs find themselves compelled to perform petty jobs in a limited arena. They discover that they are worse off than the middle-level managers in their previous organizations. And since they had never cared to learn real skills by remaining in their jobs long enough, they now find no route for escape. Which company worth its salt would like to take back a 29-year-old upstart 'CEO'? Many managerial careers have been ruined on the altar of over ambition and impatience. A tree needs time to bear fruit. But if a sapling or plant has different ideas, then only God can save it. Learn to desire only once you deserve. And to become deserving you need to spend appropriate time to equip yourself for higher responsibilities.

Before I conclude this piece, I would like to share my views on the concept of professional success with young business executives.

Now, it is not for me to tell what success should mean to you. It is a very personal and subjective issue. It is directly related to your mind and heart. It is shaped by your worldview as also the world you want to create for yourself. I, therefore, feel that managerial success cannot be and should not be measured in empirical terms. It certainly cannot be the sum of your promotions, increments, special bonuses, official commendations et al.

Success should be something far more profound and deeper. Does your managerial career satisfy you? Does your managerial work make you happy? Does your role make you feel that you are contributing to your organization, its stakeholders and society at large? Is your managerial position, at whatever level it may be, enabling you to become a more accomplished professional? Is your managerial office in sync with your personal life and goals?

If you find yourself saying 'yes' to most of these queries, then you are successful. You do not need any external signposts to announce or endorse your success.

Classical business theorists may find this definition rather bizarre. What about the balance sheet, Profit and Loss statement (P&L) account, Earnings Before Interest, Taxes, Depreciation, and Amortization (EBITDA), No Value Added (NVA), quarterly targets, production and sales figures, etc., they may ask? Little do they realize that all the above figures are mere by-products of the pursuit of excellence. And who can pursue excellence better than managers who find their work interesting, satisfying and joyful! Such managers know that the rise up the managerial ladder is but natural for them. These are the managers with wings. They are the high flyers. They are the ones who are remembered for the standards they set, the teams they built, the talent they nurtured, the missions they accomplished, the new vision they created for the company and the service they rendered to society. They are the ones who are revered in the annals of a nation's history.

Nepal needs such managers.

Preventing Corporate Burnouts

August 2017

It's a tough time for corporates the world over. The global economy is just about crawling. Growth rates are apparently in a state of semi-paralysis. The light at the end of the tunnel seems too far away.

No wonder corporate executives are battling with all their might to rekindle at least some hope for revival. In the process, they have turned into candles burning at both ends. Perhaps unknowingly, they are getting destroyed physically and mentally. The corporate world has always been a grinding place, particularly for managers who aspire to grow and excel. Success extracts its pound of flesh. Very few young executives are good at balancing work and life. Anxiety, depression, panic, etc. have become constant companions of high-flying business managers. The internal dysfunction gets manifested as hypertension, volatile blood pressure, diabetes, cardiac problems and other attendant ailments.

Burnout has become a fearsome but inevitable reality. There is no dearth of unfortunate instances when managers and CXOs in their thirties or early forties have suddenly dropped dead at their office desks. The more fortunate ones are able to scrape through long stays in hospitals. Once they emerge with their shattered body and psyche, they find themselves chained to a rigorous regimen of medication and healthcare for a lifetime.

The young manager then turns philosophical. What good, he thinks, is such success in the corporate world where the coveted corner cabin leads to the hospital ward or to a drastically truncated career? Name, fame, power, authority and wealth start appearing ephemeral. Here today, gone tomorrow. The ego takes a beating and the morale plunges into darkness. Very few emerge the same again.

The only solace seems to be the fact that the victims find this happening all around themselves. Friends and known ones in other companies and even other countries seem to be suffering the same fate. The symptoms are more or less the same everywhere. But few care to accept the fact that the root cause of the malaise is one and the same: greed, avarice and vaulting ambition to reach the top as soon as possible. The rat race is so intense that few are willing to admit that the damage they inflict upon themselves cannot be fully repaired. Over time, the sore only festers. Even the winner in the rat race remains a rat; he or she does not become a lion.

Business psychologists and organizational behaviour experts have been mulling over the issue for years. They have been recommending work – life balance and have devised several techniques. But their advice has mostly fallen on deaf ears. The exigencies of the corporate world and the race to raise the bottom line from quarter to quarter render sage advice useless. Managers have yet to understand the difference between working hard and working smart. Promoters and company top brass too cannot escape blame. They still take great pride in praising many of their 'bright stars' for working 'as hard as gadhas (donkeys)'. But one has yet to come across a donkey winning the Derby. Yet, participating in this illusory contest many donkeys break their legs and become lame for life. The ones who work smart, gallop past the winning post.

Of late, another contentious issue has cropped up in the corporate world. Does retirement at a younger age enhance a business professional's longevity? One can come across a lot of 'data' supporting this thesis in the social media and public domain. It finds easy believers also because fed up with the killing pace of corporate life many managers in their heart of hearts wish to retire as early as possible. But if you dig a little deep, you will find that such figures and claims are not rooted in reality. They are not authentic but mere hearsay.

The best-known example of such skulduggery is a so-called research paper from aircraft-maker Boeing. The paper is believed to suggest that employees who retire at 55 live to, on average, 83 years of age. But those who retire at 65 only last, on average, another 18 months. The report has been widely quoted by print and web news media. 'The problem with it,' according to the reputed BBC, 'is that Boeing itself says it's simply not true.'

On the contrary, there is a strong school of thought that those who retire late live longer. In fact, a study on its past employees in the US by the oil behemoth Shell discovered that 'mortality was slightly earlier—on average—for staff who retired at 55, than for those who continued working to 65.'

My experience as an entrepreneur and industrialist prompts me to tilt towards the above observation. Business persons or managers who remain gainfully and happily engaged in their professional activity enjoy a longer and a more fulfilling life. Many business promoters and industrialists in their eighties are still doing remarkably well in our part of the world. We need not always draw inspiration from Warren Buffet.

However, the most vital factor here is your engagement and involvement in your work, whether you are the owner or a manager. True engagement occurs when the vision and objectives of the company managers and the company are in sync. No less vital is the creation and nurturing of a work culture which keeps work-related stress in check. Promoters and owners need to realize that a person is not born just to work for a business corporation, government office or for himself. Man does not live by bread alone. He has other non-material longings and aspirations as well. Is the organization facilitating the employee to live a full and satisfying life to the best extent possible? If it is doing so, then its managers should love to be with it for long and, being relatively stress-free, also enjoy long healthy lives.

The rapidly changing business dynamics has prompted companies to alter their ways and systems. Practices like flexi-time and work-from-home are becoming increasingly popular. The core information technology industry, which offers services across oceans, has managed to keep many of its best employees in good humour by remaining in the vanguard of this change. Non-IT digital businesses too are adopting the new system with success.

Enlightened companies are gradually abandoning the command-and-control mindset. They are reposing greater trust in their executive cadre, mainly women who prefer the new system. The company too saves money on overheads like office accommodation, utility and conveyance expenses, etc. A win-win situation emerges. A happy employee is a productive employee. And productivity is the key to corporate success. Management thinker and author Stephen Covey hit the bull's eye when he stated, 'Always treat your employees exactly as you want them to treat your best customers.' Any manager worth his salt knows that acquiring a new customer is far more difficult and expensive than retaining an old one. Similarly, retaining an old employee is far more beneficial than recruiting, inducting, training and mentoring a new one. While all this is good for the organization it is equally good for its managerial cadre and other employees.

I have seen that age is more often than not a state of mind. It has little to do with the springs you have witnessed fly past. A change in our outlook, attitude and ways can make our companies and their managers remain young forever.

Upgrade Before It's Too Late

September 2017

We think we see yet we don't. What this effectively means is that though we keep hearing and reading about various developments in the world, we are rarely able to assess their impact on our lives. To be honest, we hardly bother to understand what the changing world could mean for the way we live or do business. We do accept that new developments in technology, business processes, management concepts, etc. may, sooner or later, pose new challenges for us. Yet we do not, usually, try to change ourselves at the same pace to meet those challenges. Humans are prone to thinking that bad things will happen only to others. So when the new reality starts knocking on the doors like a ravenous wolf we find ourselves at our wits' end.

Many in the world of business and its management keep their eyes open but remain blind to the obvious. They end up blaming the stars for the disaster that befalls them. But it is often too late. Many fall by the wayside. The intelligent and the aware understand, adopt, adapt and flourish. You can't beat technology. Nobody has been able to do so, so far. We have witnessed technology changing our lives since the advent of mankind. We have also seen how it made our lives easier but, in the process, also ate up jobs and livelihoods. Let's start with the invention of the wheel in ancient times. It adversely impacted the employability of trainers and attendants of horses and other draught animals like camels, elephants, oxen, etc. Because an animal-powered cart fitted with wheels could carry more people and goods than what an animal could on its back.

Moving ahead we discovered automobiles, particularly tractors and farm machines. Out went most farm animals. Major dairies no longer employ traditional milkmen. Machines milk the cows more efficiently. And the poor bulls have also been rendered largely redundant as artificial insemination is spreading fast and wide. One can only sympathize with the bulls. They are now reduced to adding some buoyancy to the stock markets. But these bulls are not of the bovine kind; they belong to the human species. What a loss for the real bulls!

The list of technological inventions can go on ad infinitum. Where are the typewriters and typists who crowded corporate offices till a decade or two ago? Secretaries of yore are gone too. They have been replaced by computer-savvy personnel. The bribe-seeking landline phone technicians have become an extinct species as mobiles turn ubiquitous.

App-based taxi aggregators are driving out individual cab owners. Banks are cutting down their staff and propelling customers towards net banking. And talking of the internet, one wistfully remembers the once eagerly awaited postman. Where has he vanished?

Cutting a long story short, I would say that automation is taking over our lives. Rapid progress in the realm of artificial intelligence (AI) is changing the face of IT. With IT governing almost all facets of business in the developed, developing and underdeveloped parts of the planet, the impact of automation and AI on jobs needs to be considered with all seriousness and sincerity. The issue can no longer be brushed under the carpet. The hungry wolf's growl is audible.

It's time we dealt with some hard data.

Labour costs are rising, even in China which grew exponentially on the back of labour arbitrage in manufacturing. To maintain and boost productivity, businesses are finding that automation is the only way out. It is an existential conundrum. Wu Ying, partner of Shanghai-based Grant Thornton, was recently quoted as saying, 'China is facing a threat to its global manufacturing status. That will be a big challenge for China to tackle over the next five to 10 years.' No wonder, China will very soon have more manufacturing robots than any other country in the world. After all, it has to compete with relatively low-wage neighbours like Vietnam, the Philippines, Thailand, etc. The government is offering special concessions to industrial units advancing towards automation. Side by side, China is also trying to produce more high value work which fetches better profits. But that could be a long haul for a country which has been used to capturing the global market share through its cheaply priced products. This calls for business process automation (BPA). High-value products need a far more mature R&D, innovation and original research lineage and large investment. Gestation periods are long. The West as also Japan is way ahead on that front. They are the real masters of technology intellectual property rights (IPRs).

However, it would be utterly misleading to suggest that BPA is only China's quest. It has become a global trend. Grant Thornton's International Business Report (IBR) based on a survey of more than 2,500 executives across 36 economies says that 56 per cent of firms are either automating processes or plan to do so over the next 12 months. Obviously some jobs will be lost, mainly in the manufacturing, technology and food and beverage sectors.

Let me quote Steve Perkins, global leader for technology at Grant Thornton: 'In this digital age, businesses are increasingly looking to technology. Post-financial crisis, firms continue to strive for greater efficiency and better productivity, and as businesses consider whether to invest in staff or machines, for many the latter is the more cost-effective solution.' It would be foolhardy on our part to assume that this trend will not catch up with us in Nepal. We are part of a globalized world. Even to do business with the outside world we will have to go in for BPA. We should also not forget that nearly 30 per cent of our gross domestic product (GDP) comes from migrant remittances. Most Nepali migrant labour is engaged in Gulf Cooperation Council (GCC) countries like Saudi Arabia, Qatar, Kuwait, etc., GCC is facing a major economic downturn because of the plunge in the prices of petroleum products, as also on account of internecine conflicts. In an unexpected move, Saudi Arabia has imposed taxes and withdrawn quite a few subsidies. Other GCC countries too are in the grip of a financial crunch. Their uncertain future has become more acute with USA starting export of crude on the back of its success in shale gas fracking. One fears that all this will eventually compel GCC countries to opt for greater automation leading to loss of jobs for Nepalese and other migrant labour. The return of our young men from foreign shores will not only upset the domestic economy but will also cause a social upheaval. Add to that the inevitable automation of industries in Nepal over the years and we find ourselves sitting on a ticking bomb.

One is reminded of the bleak job scenario described in books like *Humans Need Not Apply* by Stanford University academic Jerry Kaplan and *Rise of the Robots* by Martin Ford, software entrepreneur and celebrated author. They foresee a jobless future.

But there is a ray of hope in the concept of 'job polarization' enunciated by economists. In short, it means that automation will cause major loss in middle-level skill jobs; low and high skill jobs will not be impacted that adversely. The Nepalese may be able to save their jobs for some time because most of them are low skilled. But will low skills attract sustainable wages? Will our GDP grow? Will Nepal get out of the poverty trap?

I don't think our powers that be are even aware of the looming crisis. The government needs to wake up and join hands with the business sector to launch a skills development programme on a war footing. Let us make it easier for workers and other employees to acquire skills that would enable them to switch jobs when the automation quake hits us.

Steve Jobs' Most Urgent Job

October 2017

As I pen this piece on the legendary Steve Jobs, the most innovative tech management visionary in our lifetime, Apple has launched its latest range of products like iPhone X, iPhone 8, iPhone 8 Plus and Apple Watch 3. The world will once again be exposed to the magic of products fathered by Jobs.

One is often left wondering how one person could virtually transform the world of personal computing, animated movies, music, phones, tablet computing, retail stores and digital publishing. Imagine what more he would have done had his life not been cut short by cancer at the age of 56! But one can draw more than solace from the fact that Steve Jobs' creation, Apple, continues to be a magically mesmerizing company even six years after his demise. Isn't it time to decipher the DNA that Jobs gifted to Apple? That work culture continues to drive Apple from success to success. It is a highly demanding culture with no place for mediocrity. It is an open secret that Steve Jobs was a difficult person to work with. All seekers of perfection are.

Steve Jobs' biographer Walter Isaacson, who has authored the life stories of Henry Kissinger, Benjamin Franklin and Albert Einstein as well, enables us to vividly view Jobs' mind at work. There are lessons galore for business leaders, managers and technologists. I am picking up just a few. Though Jobs created several time-altering products, he always considered creating an enduring company like Apple his biggest achievement. An unwavering focus personified Steve Jobs. His Zen training enabled him to keep at bay all distractions which included family, colleagues, friends and even his own health and legal challenges. He was not in the business of pleasing the world at the expense of his goals and objectives. Now we can understand how he kept churning out ever superior products as long as he lived.

The narrative hitherto could easily prompt most readers to believe that Jobs lived a difficult and complex life. While that may be true, he was all for simplicity in his products. He took great pains to ensure that users of his products, whether the Macintosh or the iPad or a plethora of others, found it easy to use them. For this genius, simplicity was the ultimate satisfaction. Users and tech experts acknowledge that Microsoft Word feels primitive when compared to Apple software. To illustrate the point, let me quote Steve Jobs' biographer Isaacson: 'Jobs aimed for the simplicity that comes from conquering, rather than merely ignoring, complexity. Achieving this depth of simplicity, he realized, would produce a machine that felt as if it deferred to users in a friendly way, rather than challenging them. "It takes a lot of hard work" he said, "to make something simple, to truly understand the underlying challenges and come up with elegant solutions."'

This quote from Jobs really appeals to the poet in me. A poet has to state even the most profound emotion as simply as he can if he wishes to be understood by the common reader or listener. To reach people's hearts the poet needs to come down from his high horse. So being simple can be most difficult.

Analysing the series of successful product launches by Jobs, we realize that the master did not believe in resting on his laurels. Most of our young managers turn complacent after a minor success. The hunger to keep on winning seems to wither away. What a pity that several corporate careers die even before they blossom! Jobs believed in raising the bar all the time not only for himself but also for his colleagues. There was no place for the mediocre in his scheme of things. Instead he chose to bend the reality and made his colleagues complete tasks in four days when they wanted months to do so. This ability to push people to the pinnacle of their hidden potential came to be known as Jobs' Reality Distortion Field. Rules for lesser mortals did not apply to him and he convinced his team that those did not apply to them either.

Isaacson recalls, 'An early example was when Jobs was on the night shift at Atari and pushed Steve Wozniak to create a game called Breakout. Woz said it would take months, but Jobs stared at him and insisted he could do it in four days. Woz knew that was impossible, but he ended up doing it.'

That is how Jobs spearheaded a paradigm shift in computer history with resources which were virtually nothing in comparison to the then technology giants like IBM and Xerox. This being the background, should we perceive Steve Jobs as a maniac pursuing commercial gains? Far from it—the maestro always put products before profits.

Isaacson describes Jobs' credo so aptly: 'When Jobs and his small team designed the original Macintosh, in the early 1980s, his injunction was to make it "insanely great". He never spoke of profit maximization or cost trade-offs. "Don't worry about price, just specify the computer's abilities," he told the original team leader. At his first retreat with the Macintosh team, he began by writing a maxim on his whiteboard: "Don't compromise." The machine that resulted cost too much and led to Jobs' ouster from Apple. But the Macintosh also "put a dent in the universe," as he said, by accelerating the home computer revolution. And in the long run he got the balance right: focus on making the product great and the profits will follow. He obviously returned to Apple to scale still greater heights.'

How many companies think on these lines? An age-old metaphor for innovation runs thus: Build a better mousetrap, and the world will beat a path to your door. But few have bothered to pay heed to this piece of wisdom. Jobs did and made himself immortal. To keep bettering himself, Jobs did not hesitate from cannibalizing his own products to introduce more advanced ones—the hallmark of a truly innovative company. Instead of upgrading the original iMac incrementally, Jobs leapfrogged to an integrated system—the combination of iTunes, the iTunes Store and the iPod which transformed the music industry. The momentous success of the iPod would have made any other businessman and his company feel over the moon, with all life's work done. But not Jobs. He spurred on to forestall any danger to it from copycats. He got worried that mobile phone makers would start adding music players to their handsets. So he chose to kill the sales of his iPod by creating the iPhone. 'If we don't cannibalize ourselves, someone else will,' he said. This is what smart managers call being on the ball, 24x7x365.

Jobs always displayed tremendous foresight. But more than that, he proved his ability to execute paradigm changes in his products. He was not a mere dreamer or seer. He was a doer.

Despite being a digital creature, Steve Jobs ran a rigorous system of face-to-face interaction with his colleagues. 'There's a temptation in our networked age to think that ideas can be developed by e-mail and iChat... That's crazy. Creativity comes from spontaneous meetings, from random discussions. You run into someone, you ask what they're doing, you say "Wow," and soon you're cooking up all sorts of ideas.' Biographer Isaacson writes that Jobs had the Pixar building designed to promote unplanned encounters and collaborations.

Technology is a great tool but it can be isolating too. The tech master knew that too well. Despite his frequent brash behaviour, Jobs never ignored the human touch in his business. He created mind-boggling products for his customers always thinking that he was making them for himself. So he gave his best shot and kept the glitches out.

Learning all about Jobs' genius and contribution to business is a job in itself. However, this much should do for now.

More Out of Less—The Warren Buffett Way

November 2017

Humankind has witnessed some highly influential business tycoons, investors and management gurus straddle across the world of commerce and money. Their accomplishments have won accolades galore and helped boost the economy and employment across the globe. A few of them have transcended the boundaries of business success and have emerged as icons and idols for society at large. Their unending compassion, unmatched philanthropy and simple living have changed the lives of millions of needy and underprivileged people. They are, no wonder, viewed as messiahs by the masses.

I am about to discuss the story of a living legend. He is the world's 87-year-old leading investment guru Warren Buffett, heading his renowned organization Berkshire Hathaway. Buffett is currently the world's second richest man with a net worth of $81.1 billion. He had the distinction of being the wealthiest person in 2008 till he was overtaken by his much younger friend Bill Gates of Microsoft. And the most credible reason for the climb-down is considered to be his philanthropic donations worth billions, going among others, to the Bill & Melinda Gates Foundation. You may be surprised to know that

Buffett has pledged to allocate 99 per cent (yes 99 per cent) of his wealth for philanthropic purposes.

It is obvious that Buffett is made of a different clay. His wealth has failed to negatively impact his simplicity. The glamour and glitz of the high business world have left him untouched. He continues to live in a house bought in Omaha, Nebraska. The house has no boundary wall; it is surrounded by a hedge. Other business barons less than one-hundredth his size whiz around in luxury private jets. But Buffett still prefers to fly economy class in short flights. And, mind you, he is 87.

No wonder then that Warren Buffett's style of business has come to be known as Buffettology. It has become an academic and research discipline in itself. That is the aura of Buffett, popularly and reverentially known as the Oracle of Omaha.[9] Over 50 books, big and small, with Buffett's name in the titles have been published so far. Differently titled as *The Buffettology Workbook*, *The Tao of Warren Buffett*, and so on, these books have been translated into 17 languages and have sold more than 1.5 million copies. (Publishing circles believe that as many books have perhaps been printed only about the Dalai Lama.) However, the distinction of authoring Buffett's most credible and award-winning biography goes to Alice Schroeder.

Buffett did have his share of formal education completing his Master of Science in Economics from Columbia Business School. But the germ of investing and business had infested his system way before when he was in school. Obviously, he was not reading any tomes and treatises on the art and science of the stock market and investment. On the contrary, he drew his inspiration from Dale Carnegie's famous book *How to Win Friends and Influence People*.

Having been a salesman in the initial phase of his career, Carnegie knew his onions. He was an astute observer of consumer behaviour.

---

[9]Living and working in Omaha, Nebraska, Warren Buffett was nicknamed the 'Oracle of Omaha' due to his successful investment selections.

Buffett paid heed to his findings like few others before him. He imbibed Carnegie's observations and inferences and started practising them silently and intently. Young managers today need to follow in Buffett's footsteps. The university of life can often teach us more and better than the portals of formal academia.

The greatest entrepreneurs of current times have risen to the top of the heap this way. Being a college dropout seems to have become the in thing in the reigning high success business domain. Bill Gates, Steve Jobs, Mark Zuckerberg, Jack Ma among others were not students in the conventional mould. They had launched companies in their teens and then slogged to make them humongous. They were persons of vision. They believed in their dreams.

But much before this young lot, 1930-born Buffett had begun his act. And as I stated in a paragraph above he drew his inspiration from Dale Carnegie's commonplace observations. He discovered the kernel of human nature in them and found it worked. No wonder we still find Carnegie's magnum opus selling briskly in posh bookshops as well as with footpath book vendors. Buffett came across Dale Carnegie's famous book in his grandfather's library when he was hardly ten. Carnegie's writing made it straight to young Warren's heart which was beating hard to become a businessman. To us Carnegie's rules such as 'If you are wrong, admit it quickly and emphatically', 'Everybody wants attention and admiration. Nobody wants to be criticized' and 'Call attention to people's mistakes indirectly. Let the other person save face', etc. may sound all too obvious. But these had a profound impact on Buffett, according to his biographer, Alice Schroeder. 'Warren's heart lifted', she wrote. 'He thought he had found the truth... This was a system. He felt so disadvantaged socially that he needed a system to sell himself to people, a system he could learn once and use without having to respond in a new way to each changing situation.' Buffett returned to the book again and again for a decade. It served as the gospel for him.

Though young in years, Buffett began putting Carnegie's teachings into practice. 'People around him did not know he was performing experiments on them in the silence of his own head, but he watched how they responded… He kept track of his results. Filled with a rising joy, he saw what the numbers proved: the rules worked,' Schroeder wrote.

Without going into the intricacies of Buffett's investment deals, it is obvious that he has grown beyond the dreams of most tycoons by following simple principles of life. How else does one get to own 88 businesses and employ 233,000 workers worldwide simply by 'saving more than you borrow, making people feel good about themselves, and learning from your mistakes.' He also said, 'Businessmen may become philanthropists, but philanthropists don't become businessmen. St Francis of Assisi did not become the CEO of a global chain of bird shops.'

Buffett is known for directing key managers of his companies to write him a letter telling him who in the company would succeed them if they were to die tomorrow. These letters are updated each year. This way, if something does happen to one of his managers, time won't be wasted in trying to find a replacement.'

The multi-billionaire is known for enjoying a life with simple tastes, frugal living and generous philanthropy. However, Buffett does not describe himself as frugal but just as a man with simple tastes. 'I buy everything I want in life,' he told *People* magazine recently. 'Will 10 homes make me more happy? Possessions possess you at a point. I don't like a $100 meal as well as a hamburger from McDonald's.' He lives in the same house which he bought in 1958 for $31,500, the equivalent of roughly $270,000 at this point in time.

The Oracle's logic is simple: consider buying a smaller home than you can afford. Instead of paying pricey mortgage payments, you'll be able to put more of your money towards savings, retirement or vacations. And if you must take out a loan, consider getting a 30-

year mortgage. 'It is the best instrument in the world,' Buffett told CNBC. Buffett took out a 30-year mortgage in 1971 when he bought a vacation home in California.

'If you're wrong and rates go to 2 per cent, which I don't think they will, you pay it off,' he said. 'It's a one-way renegotiation. It is an incredibly attractive instrument for the homeowner and you've got a one-way bet.'

It should be amply clear by now why markets and investors have such immense faith in Buffett.

The Cola Lady

December 2017

When Indra Krishnamurthy Nooyi speaks, the world listens. Not just because she happens to be the chairperson and CEOof PepsiCo, the world's second largest food and beverage business. And not because she is the third wealthiest woman CEO of Fortune 500, ranking (44). Nooyi is 62 now but global captains of industry have been reverently lapping up her words of wisdom for long.

The Indian-American lady does not dabble in the nitty-gritty of business in her public speeches. That is for the treatises and tomes of business management that professors swear by. Despite having done her MBA from Yale, Nooyi has preferred to distil all her management gyan into values which make us better human beings. You can become a bloated moneybags through business trickery but you cannot become a respected business leader by pursuing money alone. You can collect hordes of gold but getting the golden shine remains the preserve of only a few.

Businessmen who transcend business considerations while remaining involved in commerce evolve into higher beings like Nooyi. The world becomes their concern. Their work becomes a passion. They work for the sheer joy of it. And they end up raising others around them. No wonder they are idolized by millions, mainly upcoming business executives, and are remembered forever. Recently I happened to come across a YouTube speech delivered by Indra Nooyi at the Rashtrapati Bhavan in New Delhi. I found it succinct and scintillating. Let me analyse the salient features of the short address.

Nooyi started off by referring to Malcolm Gladwell's 2008 bestseller *Outliers: The Story of Success*. Talking about 'outliers', that is, the most famous and successful persons in the world, Gladwell makes a very pertinent point which we often tend to overlook in our lives. Usually we try to assess what successful people are like. Rarely do we care to discover their background, that is, where are they from, their family, culture and generation, and the very different and special features of their upbringing. Referring to Gladwell's book, Nooyi told the august audience in the presence of the then President of India Pranab Mukherjee, '… who you are cannot be separated from where you came from. I left India 35 years ago, went on to the United States and went on to have tremendous success in that meritocracy. But none of that could have happened if I hadn't had a wonderful upbringing very much here in India. So I have a lot to thank India for.'

It really gladdened the hearts of Indians to find Nooyi being grateful to India despite being an American citizen now perched atop the corporate pinnacle. She broke many a ceiling to rise to such heights—being a non-white Asian, that too, a woman. These are still major handicaps even in the so-called advanced world. Nooyi performed spectacularly in the West's dog-eat-dog business world. Indeed, she does not have too many peers or competitors amongst professional managers. Nooyi shared three lessons with the listeners. You will find them very simple. But we often falter in life because we neglect the basics or consider them insignificant.

'First,' she said, 'please be a lifelong student. When we were kids, we asked questions like, why is the sky blue? Why is that bird flying so high? But for some reason as we grow, that curiosity goes away.' She cautioned the listeners that we atrophy when we become happy with the knowledge we have. Unwilling to remain a lifelong student we gradually turn into fossils. 'Don't lose that curiosity,' she urged.

What Nooyi said at the Rashtrapati Bhavan is all the more relevant today when change has become the only constant. Technology is developing at an incredible pace. Artificial intelligence is emerging both as a threat and an opportunity depending on your level of curiosity and the willingness to remain on the learning curve. Anticipating the future, using tools like big data and even sheer intuition is imperative. Complacency can kill. We have seen the debacle of world champs like Nokia and Kodak. Real estate giants are hankering for high net worth clients. Only the other day, a Dubai construction behemoth held a roadshow in Mumbai to lure customers. The plummeting fortunes of petroleum-producing countries are causing political and social upheaval in West Asia. All these companies or countries refused to see the storm staring at them and are finding themselves in a soup. Revival is terribly difficult, though not impossible. The required surgery will be painful. We can see how petro-exporter Venezuela is virtually gasping for breath. And if this can happen to the affluent West Asia and other industrial conglomerates, then we can well imagine the fate which awaits weaker economies and smaller business enterprises. So keep your eyes open, remain vigilant and keep upgrading yourself to meet new challenges. The smarter lot, whether countries, industrial groups, companies or business professionals, can turn threats and challenges into opportunities.

The second advice Nooyi offered was this: 'Whatever you do throw yourself into it. Throw your head, heart and hands into it. I look at my job, not as a job. I look at it like a calling, like a passion. I don't care about the hours. I don't care about the hardship because to me everything is a joy. So whatever you do please look upon it as a calling, as a passion, not as a job, not as something temporary.'

I find the lady's suggestion highly relevant for Nepal at this juncture. Major economic, political and social upheavals in Saudi Arabia and Qatar are ominous signs for Nepal. Over half a million Nepalese youth work as migrant labourers in these two countries alone. The situation in other countries in the region, as well as in Malaysia, is not too heartening. It is an open secret that Nepalese youth are compelled to work under difficult and at times inhuman conditions in these countries. One can only expect our embassies to protect the interests of our workers there. As of now, large-scale return is not an option. But if turmoil escalates in West Asia, then our migrant workers may be forced to come home. Considering the fact that the majority of our workers abroad hail from the Madhesh region, their return may have serious socio-political implications. Skill enhancement of potential Nepalese migrants is called for. The government needs to act expeditiously. Small and medium enterprises need to be incentivized. Modern agriculture and agri-business techniques need to be introduced to optimize the potential of the farm sector.

But how can all this happen fast enough? Through a change in mindset! Nooyi's third but most important suggestion was to help others rise:

'Greatness does not come from a position but from helping build the future. All of us in positions of power have an obligation to pull others up. As I stand here today I do not look at it as an honour but as a challenge, responsibility and an obligation to make it possible for people who are younger to come up and achieve levels of greatness.'

Easier said than done! Yet imperative!

What's Hidden in Failure?

March 2018

You learn nothing from life if you think you are right all the time. However, if you are willing to examine and analyse your failures sincerely, the road to success becomes smoother.

Young managers often marvel at the stupendous success of legendary captains of industry and tend to presume that it's all due to luck. They find it difficult to believe that business tycoons too would have encountered repeated failures and even fallen by the wayside before tasting success. In fact, even first-time big success is never permanent. To do outstandingly well in business one has to be ready to face ups and downs all the time and master the art of tackling challenges.

That is the story of almost all business barons. Let me share with you the trials and tribulations faced by some of the business icons who continue to inspire the current generation.

Many of you must have heard the name of billionaire Jack Ma who founded Chinese e-commerce site Alibaba in 1999. Forbes assessed his net worth at $36 billion last year. But are you aware that he failed to bag any job he applied for after college? And these were basic starting jobs in organizations like Kentucky Fried Chicken (KFC). Two dozen job-seekers had applied, twenty-three were absorbed, leaving only Jack Ma out.

The failure spree continued as he could not get a job in any of the thirty companies he applied to in his home town Hangzhou, China. Then he tried to join the police. There were five applicants, four got selected barring Jack. When he tried to get a waiter's job in the town's only four-star hotel, he lost out to his cousin who had scored less than him.

But Jack did not lose heart. According to CNBC's David Grogan, the early rejection taught him an important business lesson: 'You have to get used to failure,' he stated, speaking much later at the University of Nairobi. Jack Ma told an author in 2015 that he was turned down by Harvard University ten times. 'I told myself, someday I should go teach there maybe,' Jack laughed off the lapses even though he found the string of failures painful. But he was, even if unwittingly, getting prepared for a glowing entrepreneurial future. He has been quoted as saying, 'If you cannot get used to failure—just like a boxer—if you can't get used to [being] hit, how can you win?'

The initial rumble and tumble stood Jack Ma in good stead when he set up Chinese e-commerce site Alibaba in 1999 and tried to raise $5 million from venture capitalists in the USA in 2001. He met with a string of 'nos'. But steeled by his earlier failures, Jack Ma triumphed over the rejections and continued with his pursuit. He had the last laugh. Those who failed to see the merit and fortitude in Jack Ma earlier must be ruing their decision. Today Alibaba commands market capitalization of about $400 billion.

Ma, therefore, now passes around case studies about failure to colleagues at Alibaba. He says, 'When you read too many success stories, people go crazy... They think "I can be successful..." (But the truth is) when you share a lot of failure stories, you learn.'

It would be vain and foolhardy to assert that one knows no fear.

Fear is a part of life and behaviour for all living beings. In the context of this article, fear of failure in business is all the more relevant. So wouldn't it be advisable to accept this reality and devise ways to combat fear when it takes us in its grip?

The bestselling author, investor and podcast host Tim Ferriss explained his unique theory in a recent TED Talk. We know that goal-setting is an essential corporate practice irrespective of the fact whether the goals have been or are achieved by companies and their rank and file. Ferriss, instead, prepared a written exercise called fear-setting. In his TED Talk, titled 'Why you should define your fears instead of your goals', Ferriss explained that he first documents his fears, lists what may or may not happen as a result of that fear, and then writes down what he can do to prevent it. He asserted that he can trace his major successes to fear-setting because his hardest choices and biggest fears are often what he needs to do most. Elaborating in a YouTube post, he said that to succeed 'you need to fail, learn how to fail and condition yourself to fail.'

Integrity: The Secret To Lasting Success

May 2018

Integrity is missing from most realms of life today. We are left with fond but fading memories of the good old days when the gap between word and action was not so horrifying. But Generation Y, also the bulwark of the current manpower in diverse domains, is deprived of even reminiscences of a time that could inspire and guide. And that too when there is so much talk on corporate governance in management classrooms and texts. There can be no substitute for real practice.

Focused as this column is on young business managers it would be in the fitness of things to uninhibitedly locate and identify the warts inhabiting the corporate body. That will be a good initiative to pave the way for the return of integrity in business—the secret to lasting success.

One is reminded of Jon Meade Huntsman Sr's book *Winners Never Cheat: Even in Difficult Times*. Jon, who passed away at the age of 80 in February 2018, started his business in speciality chemicals almost from scratch and made it to Forbes' list of America's 100 richest persons. Jon's business touched the $12 billion mark. He forked out well over a billion dollars for different philanthropic causes, mainly cancer research. Huntsman never compromised with integrity and honesty and repeatedly proclaimed that he owed his success to integrity. He wrote, 'There are no moral shortcuts in the game of business or life. There are, basically, three kinds of people—the unsuccessful, the temporarily successful, and those who become and remain successful. The difference is character.'

Even those who do not always adhere to integrity in business do admit that it is the foundation of success. But the lure of quick money and growth often makes them stray away from the right path. But they soon realize that such success does not last and deprives them of their sleep. Bereft of integrity, business growth remains stunted. Business houses crumble.

Enron used to be the shining star of American business, worldwide. Its top management and senior executives used to boast their connections even with the US President. Enron tried to step into India by setting up a 2200 MW power project at Dabhol in Maharashtra. But Enron's penchant for wheeling-dealing led to its bankruptcy and the virtual dissolution of Arthur Andersen, one of the world's leading audit and accountancy partnerships. How the mighty fall!

While this scam broke out in 2001, the worldwide emission cheating scandal by German automobile giant Volkswagen shook the business world in 2015. The company had to spend $7.3 billion to cover the scam-related costs; its stock dipped by 17 per cent, credibility went for a six and the CEO Winterkorn resigned.

The year 2009 witnessed the downfall of Satyam Computer Services, one of India's top five IT companies. Its chairman Ramalinga Raju confessed to falsification of accounts to the tune of INR 14,162 crore. Raju was convicted and the India arm of PricewaterhouseCoopers (PwC) was fined $6 million by the US Securities and Exchange Commission for collusion. Satyam was later taken over by the Mahindra group.

The list of scams is endless and includes virtually all industries and all countries. Almost all the time, the culprits behind the scandals are the owners or the top management. They suffer ignominy, loss of their business empires, imprisonment... But they are savvy enough to stash away the ill-gotten wealth in tax havens and similar destinations which are beyond the reach of the law. Once freed, they don't have to exactly beg around for a living.

So who are the worst sufferers? None but the young business executives whose dreams go up in smoke. They flounder around to find a fresh footing. But with the rotten reputation of their fallen companies they find few takers in the job market. Corporates will not touch them even with a bargepole fearing that they will infect the new company with their dishonest work culture. The tragedy is that most young managers from tainted companies are not directly involved in scandalous business activity. Yet their career goes downhill because of their association with dirty companies. Prospective employers tend to believe that these young ones have not been exposed to the practice of integrity and corporate governance. Good companies would not like to vitiate their carefully nurtured work culture by inducting "rotten apples".

Though I would not like to name the companies concerned, I am aware of several corporates and groups in the subcontinent which continue to run on archaic and feudal patterns. So deeply entrenched are they in dishonest practices that they refuse to change their ways despite fast losing their name and worth. Not willing to approve of their management style the current generations of many such families have refused to inherit these discredited companies. They would not like to let the 'sab chalta hai' mental virus infect their modern businesses. After all, why do management gurus and leading CEOs lay so much stress on integrity? It is all about building trust—the bedrock of business or, for that matter, any other relationship. Business leaders are very careful about giving promises. But once they make the promise, they follow through on it come what may. This builds strong and reliable business-customer relationships. It becomes easier to retain old customers. New ones come driven by good word of mouth. Trust also cements the relationship between employer and employee and increases productivity. What would a company be without trustworthy and efficient HR? All other things being equal, HR is the only differentiator in today's business.

All this sums up what has come to be known as the reality principle, that is, 'seeing the world as it really is, not as you wish it to be.' Leaders with integrity are not afraid of facing the truth. They have the guts to employ people who tell them the truth on their face. They keep yes-men at an arm's distance. Many companies have perished or are on the decline because of neglecting the reality principle.

And how can a business ignore the value of integrity and transparency with the rapid rise in technology. Dishonest behaviour can be easily tracked online. We can see the predicament being faced by Facebook and Cambridge Analytica currently. Their dubious business practices have been unravelled through technology of which they themselves are the masters. What an irony!

Benjamin Franklin once observed, 'It takes many good deeds to build a good reputation and only one bad one to lose it.' Trust and integrity are indeed eternal. That is why what Franklin said in the eighteenth century rings true even today.

Communicating With Your Team Is Paramount

June 2018

How long ago did you have a heart-to-heart talk with yourself? Don't remember? Well then, how often do you really dive deep into your mind to chat with your inner self? Again unable to recall readily? Don't you find this rather embarrassing?

Well, you need not, especially if you happen to be a young and ambitious business manager. In fact, you are in the company of innumerable peers who have lost their moorings, caught as they are in the turmoil of day-to-day business data. Therefore, it is no surprise that the current crop of corporate executives is missing the woods for the trees. Mired in tackling the daily challenges of business, these youngsters fail to see the bigger picture. The holistic view is missed. Consequently, employees' engagement with the company vision and mission does not gain the requisite strength. Business suffers.

If you think deeply you will realize that there is little difference between humans and business corporations. When humans lose the connection between themselves and their souls, they tend to become rudderless. Similarly, when companies neglect internal communication their employees turn into a boat without an anchor. Such a boat sinks instantly when the waters get choppy.

Young managers must have noticed that most companies in Nepal focus largely on external communication. They use diverse ways to advertise their products or services to attract customers. They also work hard on communicating with other external stakeholders like suppliers, distributors, vendors, bankers, regulators, shareholders in case of public companies, etc. Compared to this, scant attention is paid to communicating with company employees. The top management still believes in the archaic command-and-control system. Against this backdrop, how can the rank and file of the company have their heart in its growth and prosperity? Will they go out of their way to come up with novel suggestions to improve the organization's performance? How can they when there is no systematic process to encourage horizontal and vertical, particularly bottom-up, communication.

Enlightened companies in the world have realized the significance and virtue of internal communication to enhance employee engagement. They implement elaborate schemes to make their employees feel an integral part of the company's decision-making. The CEB/Gartner's Internal Communications Summit held in November last year highlighted the corporate world's changing attitude towards the strategic importance of internal communication. A release issued on the occasion quoted research scientists Peter Weill and Stephanie L. Woerner in their 2015 MIT Sloan Management Review saying, 'Most of the productivity increase seen in organizations nowadays originates—directly or indirectly—from digitization and big data analytics...the future of internal communication should be determined by the needs of future employees.' The attendees felt that a centralized digital workplace is a 'core pillar of fostering employee engagement'.

Based on reports that in the western world corporate employees spend 80 per cent of their time on mobile devices using an app, the Summit participants inferred a widespread adoption of mobile workplace tools which would enable employees to instantly access company news, operation tools, workflows, communication channels, etc. Corporate CXOs expect that mobile communication apps will promote real-time or, at least, timely responses. With decision-making gaining pace, the overall speed of doing business will increase. There will be fewer bottlenecks. Resolution of problems will happen faster as the top management will be in the loop and provide its valuable inputs. Just a mobile phone can help employees achieve so much.

No less important is the spurt in employee engagement which usually follows increased focus on internal communication. Implemented in right earnest, internal communication turns young managers proactive and more involved in organizational affairs. After all, the best ideas are not the monopoly of the top management. Useful ideas can emanate from all levels of employees. In fact, more practical and relevant suggestions come from managers posted on the production shop floor, in the field interacting with direct customers and distribution channels, procuring and managing raw material, etc. Often their advice is no less vital than the strategic thinking at the top. Tactical inputs form the bedrock of strategic decisions. So companies need to ensure that the movement of information between the two levels is regular and timely. The Gartner's Summit observed, '... employee engagement leads to a rich company culture, a vested commitment to the success of colleagues, and a sense of pride working for a brand that cares about its people.' But this is easier said than done.

It has often been observed that middle-level management proves to be the biggest stumbling block in the implementation of internal communication. Middle managers draw their power and authority by holding on to information. Transparent and democratic flow of information breaks their hold on younger managers. No wonder, many western companies got rid of middle managers during the global meltdown. In fact, the process had begun much earlier during the dot.com bust in early 2000. The exercise came to be known as 'delayering' in management jargon. The middle-level layer was done away with as it had lost its utility. Only decision-makers and implementers remained. The trend is gradually creeping to the non-West corporate world as well, though with less force and momentum. But one cannot stall a movement whose time has come. Either the middle management will have to change in keeping with the new corporate changes, or it will have to make way for younger managers who are amenable to the new business reality.

Company biggies need to put their heads together to promote internal communication. It is time to enhance intra-company communication using new digital tools and technologies to 'encourage productivity, community, and mutual respect among' the entire workforce. Communication technologies like Search Engine Optimization (SEO) and Search Engine Marketing (SEM) are increasing and growing by the day. Therefore, companies need to spend time and resources to refresh and perfect web copy, meta tags and back-links. This is all the more important for those engaged in e-commerce.

The Gartner's release made another vital observation when it stated: 'Whereas digital experience platforms will become an increasingly important fixture for ensuring employee engagement, maintaining a traditional CMS or intranet hub will continue to be a tried and true method to host more static company assets.' This gives rise to feelings which are more lasting than what one might have heard or done. However, a company should embark on project internal communication only when it is ready to remain on its toes and keep its communication tools and content updated and fresh. Otherwise, all that goes in the name of internal communication remains a one-time ritual. Unfortunately, that is the case in most companies in our part of the world!

Businesses Need Gender Diversity

August 2018

With millions of young Nepali males serving as menial migrant labourers abroad and contributing around 32 per cent of the country's GDP in the form of remittances it is obvious that Nepali women at home are in no way behind in contributing to the country's economy. One cannot assert that womenfolk are doing this willingly but they are indeed toiling to keep home and hearth alive. With most able-bodied males compelled to work abroad in view of Nepal's precarious economic situation, women have to pitch in. Their involvement is diverse—from the agricultural sector to micro and small businesses to NGOs and INGOs.

Some women from the elite section of society do manage middle and major businesses which they have inherited. However, examples of self-made major businesses owned and run by women remain few and far between in Nepal. But this is not surprising in a largely patriarchal and feudal society.

Though the country is currently run by a communist government, it seems that a fair dispensation for our women is not foreseeable in the near future. Deeply entrenched and archaic social mores, mindset and attitude do not easily make way for a pragmatic, progressive and enlightened outlook. To some extent, Nepal shares this predicament with many of its neighbouring countries and non-western nations. We are continuing with our orthodox ways at our own peril. Women usually form half the population of any country. But in Nepal, they are all the more predominant, population-wise, as millions of our young and middle-aged males eke out a living abroad and send money home. This is our compulsion.

Should we not try to induct more women in our businesses and industries? Should we not ensure that women employees and managers are assessed and promoted solely on the basis of their competence and ability? Why should gender come in the way of their rise? Why should the glass ceiling inhibit the growth of women alone?

Nepal desperately needs diversity in its corporate rank and file. By denying women their due in the world of commerce, Nepal is depriving itself of its home-grown talent. It would be foolhardy to depend on highly paid expatriates until and unless there is an emergency and local talent in a particular domain is simply not available. We can gradually build capacity by training our own female citizens.

Though I am, in this chapter, focusing on inclusion of only women in Nepalese business and industry, it would not be out of place to quote a McKinsey report which highlights a more holistic approach on hunting and nurturing talent. The McKinsey report states: 'Our latest research analyses more data from more companies than ever before. Three years on (2018), does the link between company financial performance and ethnic, cultural, and gender diversity stand up to greater scrutiny? ... We know intuitively that diversity matters. It's also increasingly clear that it makes sense in purely business terms. Our latest research finds that companies in the top quartile for gender or racial and ethnic diversity are more likely to have financial returns above their national industry medians. Companies in the bottom quartile in these dimensions are statistically less likely to achieve above-average returns. And diversity is probably a competitive differentiator that shifts market share toward more diverse companies over time.'

It is obvious that more diverse workforces perform better financially. Some of the findings in McKinsey's report 'Diversity Matters', which are relevant to this article, examined proprietary data sets for 366 public companies across a range of industries in Canada, Latin America, the United Kingdom, and the United States. The focus was on financial results and the composition of top management and boards. The findings were clear: companies in the top quartile for gender diversity are 15 per cent more likely to have financial returns above their respective national industry medians. Companies in the bottom quartile both for gender and for ethnicity and race are statistically less likely to achieve above-average financial returns than the average companies in the dataset (that is, bottom quartile companies are lagging rather than merely not leading).

Racial and ethnic diversity has a stronger impact on financial performance in the United States than gender diversity, perhaps because earlier efforts to increase women's representation in the top levels of business have already yielded positive results. In the United Kingdom, greater gender diversity on the senior-executive team corresponded to the highest performance uplift: for every 10 per cent increase in gender diversity, EBIT (earnings before income and taxes) rose by 3.5 per cent. While certain industries perform better on gender diversity and other industries on ethnic and racial diversity, no industry or company is in the top quartile on both dimensions.

The McKinsey data provides enough pointers pertaining to benefits of gender diversity in the middle and higher echelons of the corporate world. It is a pity that such data is conspicuous by its absence in Nepal. It is also indicative of the fact that our companies are not even thinking in this direction. Barring family-run companies, I have hardly come across any women in senior management let alone the board of directors. Women continue to work largely as stenographers, telephone operators, personal secretaries and similar positions. Ironically, this is all the more so in bigger and established companies where males prevail.

Start-ups and smaller outfits, which are more exposed to the new economy, are prone to ignore gender discrimination. Run mostly by the younger generation, companies engaged in ITeS, digital marketing, advertising, designing, education, tuitions, food and beverage, trading, chartered accountancy, etc. are staunchly opposed to gender discrimination and inducting more and more women. Merit seems to be the sole criterion for employing youth—women or men.

I have rarely come across more sturdy women than the Nepalese. With a large number of able-bodied males working abroad, these girls and women hold things together in Nepal. They engage in agriculture and farm-related activities in the most difficult of terrains, run bazaar shops and markets in towns and hinterland in the face of male tyranny at home and outside. They are our real fighters, holding the fort both at home and outside. They have been multi-tasking much before the term found its way in management jargon. And, when bored, many of them scale the Everest — once, twice! All this requires both physical and mental strength and prowess.

Yet, Nepal's big business refuses to train women adequately and accommodate them in accordance with their abilities. Why this resistance to women's inclusion? When will we witness a Nepalese woman professional heading a known and reputed company in the country. When will we create an ecosystem which will encourage and motivate our women to move up the corporate ladder? Perhaps when our males get rid of their false egos! Will that happen sooner than later or ever at all?

Adversity Is the Best Teacher

September 2018

Young corporate managers must have seen the changes which passenger car or two-wheeler companies have had to undergo for sheer survival. Original and integrated equipment manufacturers in the automobile domain have to always remain on their toes to cater to the changing tastes and needs of buyers. This demands the highest level of customer awareness, ability to incorporate changes and innovation in products and services, considerable capital expenditure, etc. I am not in the auto business but do have friends and kin actively involved in this industry across the world. Seeing them work, I have started believing that a stint, the longer the better, in the auto business can serve as the best training ground for aspiring, ambitious and young executives.

The reason is simple. There is no business activity which is left untouched by an automobile company. An auto professional thus evolves as a well-rounded manager capable of tackling diverse challenges of the business. However, it is obvious that a young and middle-level executive will not be able to serve in all departments of an automobile company. But if she or he has fire in the belly, then s/he will be exposed to diverse facets of business, whether it be different aspects of manufacturing, materials management, supply chain management, import-export, technology acquisition, quality control, marketing, sales, customer surveys, research and development (which may also include reverse engineering), finance, interaction with government, bankers and regulatory agencies, internal and external communications, HRD,... the list is endless. Ancillaries have also to be dealt with. So, you see, there is a lot to learn and imbibe.

Also, the scale at which automobile companies operate is truly humongous. That is why the automobile industry is seen as the index of a country's economy. There used to be a time when it was said that if General Motors (GM) is doing well, then the USA economy is doing well. Such was the unbreakable bond between the world's biggest automobile company and the world's largest economy.

But how fickle are the fortunes of the largest corporates! Good times do not last forever if you do not work hard enough when the sun is shining. GM went bankrupt on 1 June 2009, with assets of $82.99 billion and debt amounting to $172.81 billion. How the mighty fall! Revival involved Herculean efforts but the ups and downs still continue. An almost dying Chrysler Corporation was revived by the legendary Lido Anthony Iacocca almost from ground up. He was wooed from Ford. He slogged all through the 1980s introducing new vehicles which caught people's fancy and created astonishing sales records. Having crushed the crisis and put Chrysler back on the profitable path, Iacocca retired as the company's chairman in December 1992. His advertising campaign for Chrysler cars included unforgettable slogans like 'The pride is back' and 'If you can find a better car, buy it'. However, Chrysler went bankrupt in 2009. Good times, as I stated, are not forever, if you are not on your toes 24x7.

Closer home, the maker of the iconic Ambassador, Hindustan Motors Ltd (HM) pulled down shutters in May 2014 after a 76-year run. A car of the Indian elite for decades, the Ambassador faded into oblivion as the company cared little to upgrade its technology and service standards. The very late entry of Maruti Suzuki was perceived with apathy and arrogance by HM, leading to its demise. Though many foreign brands had entered the Indian auto market by then, the Ambassador's exit was the end of an era. Its absence is still lamented by its innumerable fans, both in India and abroad. In fact, the Ambassador was adjudged the world's best taxi in a race competition conducted by BBC in the UK just a year before HM shut shop. The car used to be sturdy as a battle tank. However, the HM management forgot that customer tastes and needs had changed. People wanted small and high mileage cars, not battle gladiators. Enter Maruti in the early 1980s with its 800cc car and India witnessed a mobility revolution. In the beginning, the Maruti could not boast the sturdiness, spaciousness, comfort, elegance and prestige of the Ambassador. But ultimately economy prevailed and the middle class moved over to the affordable Maruti 800 and its later descendants. Today, Maruti Suzuki occupies 50 per cent of India's passenger market segment. Hyundai is a distant runner-up. Other global biggies like Toyota, Renault, Nissan, Datsun, Honda, Audi, Jaguar, Land Rover, BMW, Mercedes-Benz, Ford, Fiat, Skoda, Volkswagen, Tata Motors, Mahindra & Mahindra, etc. are way behind. This effectively means that barring Maruti Suzuki, most passenger car companies in India are either in the red or making minimal profits. The titan GM called it a day last year. Notably, foreign giants making profit in India owe it to exports from their units here. They have little to crow about their domestic sales. For example, Ford's total revenue from India stood at $3.1 billion last year. But domestic sales accounted for only one-third of it. Ford's India sales grew by a measly 1 per cent in 2017 at 87,588 units, while exports clocked a healthy jump of 15 per cent at 175,196 units.

One could, therefore, say that the passenger car industry too is as fickle and unpredictable as the aviation industry, especially as more and more players are venturing into these domains with novel products, revenue models and service standards. The competition is only growing even as weaklings fall by the wayside. The unstoppable expansion of social media has made businesses more vulnerable to crises. Word spreads like fire. Remember the recent recall of eight million vehicles by Toyota after a customer issue in the USA. Similarly, the emission scam by Volkswagen put the German auto behemoth on the mat and did massive damage to its carefully nurtured image.

What does this effectively mean for managers seeking a bright future in the passenger automobile industry? They should be daring enough to face frequent crises. Still better would be the ability to remain proactive and avoid crises. But strangely enough, we see the elephant only when it has entered the room, all set to trample us. Otherwise, how does one explain auto giants going bankrupt?

While there are a myriad ways to face a crisis, I feel corporate communications or public relations serve as the immediate tool when the tsunami strikes. While Coombs and Holladay have done acclaimed work in this field, a much younger Aaron Shardey, who graduated with a first class honours degree in public relations from the London College of Communications, also focused on crisis management in general. Shardey's findings rise above the Anglo-American construct and therefore have greater and wider applicability. Here are some of the salient points highlighted by him.

Preparation for situations that could occur: This was deemed vitally important, with tools and processes in place to monitor and record issues that could potentially escalate into a local and/or global (crisis) situation... issues and crisis situations arise in specific contexts; generic case studies of good and bad practice are of limited value. Instead, the value of reflection and evaluation after an incident is essential.

Organizational structure: Cross-departmental communications within and across national and global operations were revealed to require two-way processes rather than a top-down one. The importance of public relations as an integrated, strategic function operating as one department globally was reinforced. This included ensuring that internal communications are not neglected.

Cultural sensitivities: The impact of how people communicate and deal with problems in different cultures was considered, including how a corporate head office culture needs to recognize local needs within the mainstream and digital media system, and the political and legal system.

Common planning approaches: The results showed that global and local crisis management plans were deployed from global headquarters for regional operations to adopt and adapt. The necessity of a global plan is essential given the speed at which a local crisis can quickly become global, yet challenges remain in the values and cultures of specific countries. The status of the organization—and its brands—within individual countries and globally was also felt to be a key factor in local adaptation.

Shardey's four points mentioned above can serve young managers well while dealing with crises, especially in the auto sector.

Godspeed!

Marketing Tips From Superheroes

December 2018

What shall we marvel at now? Stan Lee, the legendary creator of comic characters like Spider Man, X-Men, Thor, Iron Man, the Fantastic Four, the Incredible Hulk, the Ghost Rider, Black Panther and many more, breathed his last on 12 November at the age of 95.

Lee, who influenced American popular culture in substantial measure, left behind the billion-dollar Marvel universe, comprising comic books, films, TV shows, games, digital media and merchandise. It was a magical world beyond comparison which held young and old in thrall. His peers could hardly match him.

Why was this? Because while his competitors created superheroes, Lee created characters with a human touch. Like us, Lee's characters had flaws and shortcomings. Despite being endowed with super-human powers, Lee's creations cried and wept, battled with common problems like us and were often made to even bite the dust or were humiliated. Very much like our divine avatars who faced troubles and tribulations for the ultimate good of mankind. That is what makes us believe in them. Writer Rachel Lopez commented, 'Relatable, fallible heroes were a Stan Lee signature... Other signatures Lee leaves behind:

superheroes who came from actual spots on the map, the notion that characters could cross over and team up, and heroes and villains who have often been reflective of larger social narratives.'

No wonder then millions or maybe billions of Lee's fans around the world identified themselves with these characters. And this is what gave Lee an edge over his competition. In fact, for decades, Lee had no clue about his winning gambit. Lending his superheroes a human touch came naturally to him. The competition realized the 'secret' too late. Chuckling in a TV interview, Lee once said that this proved to be a boon for the Marvel universe.

Some of his observations give an insight into his comic characters. Here they are:

With great power comes great responsibility.

- The power of prayer is still the greatest ever known in this endless eternal universe.
- That person who helps others simply because it should or must be done and because it is the right thing to do is indeed without a doubt a real superhero. *Excelsior!*
- Another definition of a hero is someone who is concerned about other people's well-being, and will go out of his or her way to help them—even if there is no chance of a reward.

But why am I talking of the comic world Czar in a management column? What management-specific lessons does Stan Lee's life offer to young managers and executives?

Didn't I refer to the human touch which was so obvious in Lee's superheroes? While it could be true that this approach may not have been deliberately devised by Lee, yet it was very much a part of his characters. One could say that this was ingrained in Lee's psyche and inadvertently found its way into his creative world. His characters became more believable among the legions of his readers and viewers.

Here is the hidden lesson for our sales and marketing executives.

Lee's work touched a chord in the customer's heart. He knowingly or unknowingly made his customers believe in his superheroes. He imbued his characters with superpowers but also made them feel and falter like humans. No fairy tales from Lee.

Do our sales and marketing staff go out of their way to map out the psychographics and demographics of our existing and potential customers? Do we try to gain a deep insight into their likes and dislikes? Do we track the changing trends and keep creating and introducing products and services accordingly? Are we willing to accept that even the best of products will fail to hold customers' fancy forever and, therefore, changes and innovations need to be introduced regularly?

Marketing is all about touching the heart. Then the sought-after appropriate sales figures will bounce upwards automatically.

Emotions Can Grow Your Business

January 2019

People generally believe that persons with a high intelligence quotient (IQ) are bound to make it big in life. That is why we lay so much stress on academic success. Parents strive to ensure that their children score the highest possible marks in tests and exams. The fascination for fancy marks often puts immense pressure on students. Unable to cope with the expectations of family and peers many youngsters burn out early in life and lose interest in studies.

With educational competition getting fiercer by the day, young people find it more and more difficult to first get admissions in the institutions or courses of choice and later, get jobs they aspire for. It is indeed painful to find that, unable to face the pressure, many youth even commit suicide. Yet our IQ-focused education and exam system continues as ever.

On the other hand, I and many of my industrialist friends, who have been recruiting and employing young managers over the decades, have detected the fallacy in the IQ-centric exams and recruitment. In fact, there is no dearth of successful professionals and businessmen who have made it to the top without having topped academic tests and exams. Are we not aware of the likes of college dropouts like Bill Gates, Steve Jobs, and not so academically brilliant business tycoons like Warren Buffett, Indian Warren Buffett Rakesh Jhunjhunwala, Dhirubhai Ambani, Jack Ma of Alibaba fame and scores of start-up entrepreneurs around the globe who have made their mark in business without having scored great marks in school or college? On the contrary, those employed by these mega achievers are often really brainy people whose marksheets are worth their weight in gold.

It is, therefore, obvious that there is something more than mere intelligence or IQ that ensures unprecedented growth and rise of individuals. What is that missing ingredient which makes the difference between professional managers and creators of massive wealth and employment? It is emotional intelligence, generally termed as emotional quotient (EQ) in management parlance.

According to Salovey and Mayer (1999), 'Emotional intelligence is the ability to perceive emotions; to access and generate emotions so as to assist thought; to understand emotions and emotional knowledge; and to reflectively regulate emotions so as to promote emotional and intellectual growth.' This can be accepted as a fairly scientific definition.

Though the precise benefits of EQ have made it to the academic world relatively recently, business tycoons with insight into human behaviour have always understood and realized their significance. They knew that the heart often rules over the head and makes people extra productive. In fact, one has witnessed emotions being the driving force over millennia in fields as diverse as global exploration, trade, commerce, management, science and technology, war, geo-politics, etc. When we talk of EQ today, we evaluate its use to increase employee engagement, improve the bottom line and promote teamwork. EQ has been found to be effective on all fronts.

Industry reports inform how in a six-month leadership development process at Komatsu Multinational Corporation, using the 'Six Seconds' Vital Signs framework, engagement increased from 33 to 70 per cent while plant performance also increased by 9.4 per cent. Kabushiki-gaisha Komatsu Seisakusho manufactures construction, mining, and military equipment, as well as industrial equipment like press machines, lasers and thermoelectric generators. In 2012 Komatsu partnered with Six Seconds to increase the engagement of people in order to build competitive capability and create a case demonstrating their commitment to innovation. The project blended assessments, training, and project-based learning to involve managers in creating a climate for innovation. According to much-chronicled industry data, this innovative approach to engaging employees led to three key findings:

Create change by letting people change: Involve the managers in a new way of thinking and working, provide them with insights and tools to experiment with alternatives.

Build teams intelligently: Powerful, innovative teams have a mix of styles, talents, EQ skills, and capabilities.

Create choice: When people self-select, they have power. They become more committed to the process, and they feel ownership of the results.

The project blended assessments, training and project based learning to involve managers in creating a climate for innovation.

People engagement was measured with Team Vital Signs (TVS), a statistically reliable research process designed to pinpoint areas assisting and interfering with growth and bottom-line success. There are five key drivers in the Vital Signs Model. A high performing team climate is driven by these five factors:

Trust: People have a sense of safety and assurance so they'll take risks, share, innovate, and go beyond their own comfort zones.

Motivation: People need to feel energized and committed to doing more than the minimum requirement.

Change: Employees and the institution are adaptable and innovative.

Teamwork: People collaborate and communicate with one another to take on the challenges.

Execution: Individuals are both focused and accountable.

The experience gained by Six Seconds, a global network supporting people to create positive change everywhere, shows that the skills of EQ are invaluable for leading change. The changes are there for all to see.

- The US Air Force saved $2,760,000 in recruitment spending due to their nominal investment (of less than $10,000) in emotional competence testing.
- According to Boyatzis (1999), consulting partners who showed high EQ earned 139 per cent more than partners with lower EQ.
- Management researchers Pesuric & Byhan wrote in 1996 that raised EQ levels cut accidents in a manufacturing plant by 50 per cent, formal grievances by 80 per cent and raised the top line by $250,000.

Does all this mean that intelligence has no place in business? The *HBR* clarifies the issue: 'The most effective leaders are alike in one crucial way: they all have a high degree of emotional intelligence. It's not that IQ and technical skills are irrelevant, they do matter, but mainly as "threshold capabilities"; that is, they are the entry-level requirements for executive positions. But research shows clearly that without emotional intelligence a person can have the best training in the world, an incisive, analytical mind, and an endless supply of smart ideas, but he still won't make a great leader.'

Businesses are fast realizing that to grow rapidly and tackle challenges, they need leaders and not mere managers. It is often said that leaders are born, not trained. But advances in management education and in-house training have shown that leadership skills can be imparted and imbibed.

To accomplish this objective, promoters and top management need to display EQ first by displaying a large heart and offering suitable opportunities to their young and middle-rung executives to utilize EQ more often. This will lead to creation of internal capacity and EQ will become a part of the company's business ethos.

Loneliness at the Workplace

March 2019

The world today abounds with ironies. How else can we explain the growing loneliness despite being digitally connected more than ever? Thanks to rapid strides by communication technology one can get in touch with anyone across continents and oceans at the click of a button. Yet loneliness and its impact on mental health are haunting even the business world.

This grave concern was echoed by the World Economic Forum at Davos this January. A report presented there warned that the global mental health crisis could cost the world $16 trillion by 2030. This will not only lower business efficiency, productivity and economic growth but will also drastically impair our social fabric. The report authored by Elisha London, CEO, United for Global Mental Health, and Peter Varnum, Project Lead, Global Health and Healthcare, World Economic Forum, states, 'Loneliness and isolation affect many of the most vulnerable among us. People with serious conditions such as schizophrenia or bipolar disorder are especially likely to be marginalized by their communities. Those with the most severe conditions pay with their lives, dying prematurely—as much as two decades before their time.'

Persons at the highest levels in the government, private sector and civil society have taken cognizance of the daunting challenge and are discussing ways to overcome it. All over the world, business leaders and management researchers are putting their heads together to devise appropriate and geography-relevant work culture changes. Efforts at the community level are no less important as mental health cannot be compartmentalized into home and workplace. Both are inextricably linked. Loneliness and isolation can afflict one both at home and office. Vulnerability to a sense of being socially abandoned is equal in severity at both the places.

There is no doubt that technological progress has made our lives easier and comfortable in many ways. But the hyperconnection to such a large number of tech devices has also added to stress, loneliness and anxiety. A 2010 report by the American Association of Retired Persons (AARP) has found that loneliness has doubled since the 1980s. Over 40 per cent of adults in America are said to feel lonely. The human touch is missing. Relationships with kith and kin have broken down and technology is unable to compensate for that loss. EuroHeartCare 2018, which is the European Society of Cardiology's annual congress, revealed that loneliness can be a strong 'predictor of dying too soon'. Loneliness is a debilitating factor at the workplace as well. The AARP report states, 'Loneliness and feeling isolated at work can lead to decline in productivity due to mental and emotional exhaustion.' After all, people spend one-third of their lives at work.

However dire and threatening all this sounds, things are not beyond redemption. There are ways to change the corporate DNA. It is not rocket science either. Consistent and caring HRDpractices can usher in significant positive changes. The HR team needs to ensure that there are opportunities for new connections during the pre-hire and post-hire process. Most employees, both managerial and staff level, do feel a sense of anxiety before joining a new company. A well-documented process of connectedness should be in place even before the new employee agrees to join. The potential new hire will feel far less isolated if he is fully briefed about the company culture and also introduced to members of the team informally. Once the person has joined, he should be given time to interact with his colleagues at group lunches and similar events. The corporate communications team should provide to the new entrant a comprehensive dossier carrying both hard and soft facts about the organization as per the need and demand of his position which will make him feel more engaged and connected.

It would be obvious from the above description that work culture should be rooted in empathy and compassion. If the culture honestly aims at promoting high performance, then focus should be on respectfulness, honesty, support and empathy. Empathy is known to prevent burnout and work exhaustion—so common in the current ultra-competitive corporate world. Research published in 2014 by Jane Dutton, co-author of *Awakening Compassion at Work,* came to the conclusion that compassion could be a key tool in fostering improved levels of workplace resiliency.

Are your employees enjoying doing their job? Or do they feel like they've fallen in a rut? This needs to be assessed as soon as possible and rectified. Efficient and effective working is important but so is enjoying the job. Routine and mundane work saps energy and dedication to work. HR managers of enlightened companies, therefore, pay a lot of attention to formal and informal group activities, mostly outside office. This not only rejuvenates the mind and heart but also bolsters team spirit, a perfect antidote to loneliness. Working managers today also expect the company to arrange training and mentoring to help them remain on top of the learning curve. Innovation and out-of-the-box thinking need to be encouraged and rewarded.

To keep your spirits high you need to keep your physique fit and robust. The two go great together. Therefore top managements should ensure that their rank and file work smart and not too hard. A good employee will be able to accomplish his task in time. Overtime working is symbolic of inefficiency. It is also a drain on the office resources in more ways than one. Can a sleepy-eyed manager, who worked overtime yesterday, put in his best today? And what if this becomes a routine? His physical well-being will go for a toss. The brain too will not be spared. Prioritization of work needs to be promoted. It should become second nature for managers. Sports and entertainment will add to wellness.

Here I would like to quote United States Surgeon General Vivek H. Murthy, who stated the following in the *HBR*: 'If we cannot rebuild strong, authentic social connections, we will continue to splinter apart—in the workplace and in society. Instead of coming together to take on the great challenges before us, we will retreat to our corners, angry, sick, and alone. We must take action now to build the connections that are the foundation of strong companies and strong communities—and that ensure greater health and well-being for all of us.'

It is thus obvious that social connection is a key factor in contributing to the company's bottom line. Let's build and nurture this bond.

Sustainable Business

April 2019

The United Nations' report 'Sixth Global Environmental Outlook' released mid-March sends a chill down the spine. Prepared by 250 scientists and experts from over 70 countries, the report states that millions of early deaths will occur by year 2050 if we fail to tackle the growing challenges to the environment. Cities and regions in Asia, the Middle East (West Asia) and Africa will bear the brunt of this blow, the report asserts.

Urgent action is called for to protect people's health. It is obvious the most grievously affected will be those occupying the lowest rung on the social ladder.

The report warns that 'pollutants in the fresh water systems will see anti-microbial resistance become a major cause of death by 2050 and endocrine disruptors impact male and female fertility, as well as child neurodevelopment.'

With more and more people meeting a premature end and fertility being affected adversely, mankind will be gradually heading towards extinction. Children with inadequate neurodevelopment will turn out to be a burden on their families and society. The relationship between a fast deteriorating environment and human health will become more and more fearsome and frightful.

The idea is not to create a scary scenario but to caution all about what may happen if we continue to remain complacent. There is however, a reassuring part to this situation in that things are not beyond redemption yet. The UN report too states that all is not lost. The world has enough scientific, technological and financial resources to develop and practise a model of sustainable development. Incidentally, people, business and political leaders have still not developed the vision to realize this. They are still striving for short-term gains. As for the youth, it is enamoured by instant gratification. The environment cannot suffer this predatory attitude beyond a point. There will come a point when the balance is broken and it will be compelled to react in the form of climate change leading to natural disasters, like the rise in temperatures which we are already seeing. This alone makes glaciers, oceans, mountains, etc. go haywire. The devastation caused is unimaginable. Haven't we heard enough about the trail of devastation left by typhoons, tsunamis, unpredictable floods and droughts, snow avalanches, drying rivers and waterbodies, unbreathable air, choking smogs, etc.? And even the advanced and rich countries are not spared from these extreme natural events. After all, they were the pioneers in environment destruction. Their smoke-belching factories robbed our air of its pristine purity and turned many of our cities into virtual gas chambers. This is both noxious and obnoxious.

What role can the business world play in protecting the planet from further degradation and initiating a healing and restorative process? First and foremost, we need to ensure that our managers, particularly the younger lot, are made aware of the repercussions of neglecting and harming the environment. One cannot continue with outdated production systems and still expect nature to remain benevolent towards us. How can Mother Earth do much for us when we have ourselves polluted its oceans, rivers and lakes and poisoned its air? It is wounded and crying.

Our managers need to abandon outmoded and traditional approaches and adopt innovation with fervour. The first objective should be to replace fossil fuels—that is, coal and petroleum products—with hydroelectricity to run our factories and vehicles. Hydroelectricity can become Nepal's major strength and a game changer for its economy. Electric mobility is picking up the world over. Solar energy also needs to be promoted. One can draw a lesson from Morocco which is successfully scaling up solar energy. The kingdom proposes to become a powerhouse of renewable energy and export electricity to Europe in a few years' time.

The UN's bid to turn the planet healthy is based on changing the 'grow now, clean up after' model to a near-zero-waste economy by the year 2050. According to the Global Environmental Outlook, green investment of 2 per cent of countries' GDPs would deliver long-term growth as high as the presently projected but with fewer impacts from climate change, water scarcity and loss of ecosystems. The report advises adopting less meat-intensive diets and reducing food waste in both developed and developing countries, as it would reduce the need to increase food production by 50 per cent to feed the projected 9–10 billion people on the planet in 2050. Strategic investment in rural areas can reduce pressure on people to migrate. Attention has been drawn to the need to curb the flow of the 8 million tonnes of plastic pollution going into oceans each year. But there is still no global agreement to tackle marine litter. Thankfully, the UN report shows that policies and technologies already exist to fashion new development pathways that will avoid these risks and lead to health and prosperity for all people. What is needed is a strong will to act on the part of politicians and big business.

Business promoters and managers need to realize that going beyond business activities and taking care of the environment can bring business benefits. Now corporate companies have understood that business activity in an environmentally friendly way is not only a legal duty but also a responsibility. Although Nepal seems to be lagging behind in this respect, stakeholders all over the world increasingly require corporate organizations to become more environmentally aware and responsible. No wonder, CSR (corporate social responsibility) has become more focused and is known as CER—corporate environmental responsibility. Earlier in the traditional business model, environmental protection had been considered only in relation to 'public interest', but now it's a part of business. So the synergy between business and environmental responsibility is growing stronger in enlightened companies. In Nepal, younger managers, who are more aware about the business-environment bond, need to take the lead.

Experts have listed several environment conservation methods such as: safe and secure storage of waste, its appropriate treatment, collection by an authorized body such as your local municipal authority or a licensed waste contractor, managing waste for recycling by separating paper, plastic, metals and glass and for those organizations that are in the food businesses, separation of food waste for recycling.

Managers need to take care that their business activities do not cause a statutory nuisance like production of smoke, noise, gases, odour, fumes, and accumulation of rubbish or light pollution which are injurious to health. In case business activities pose an imminent threat to the environment, then managers need to notify the relevant enforcing body to take steps to prevent the damage. Managers need to be extra careful about the risks posed by chemicals or hazardous substances like oil, chemicals, pesticides, ozone-depleting substances, radioactive materials, electrical or electronic equipment solvents and biocides. Use of certain hazardous substances such as lead, mercury and calcium, usually in the manufacturing sector, should be handled with caution. Managers should prevent placing products on the market with more than a certain amount of hazardous substances.

Similarly, extra attention needs to be paid to equipment containing ODS (Ozone Depleting Substances) or fluorinated gases. Checking for leakages and record-keeping for recycling should form part of the managers' regimen.

Conservation of biodiversity includes all species of animals (wildlife) and plants. Increasing human activities cause loss of biodiversity and this needs to be prevented. This not only applies to land-based industries such as farming and forestry but also to all factories, industries, offices and other business activities based on or near biodiversity areas.

Managers have a lot on their platter. They need to pay immediate attention to all responsibilities so that business and the environment thrive together.

Ambition Is a Double-edged Sword

May 2019

The line dividing aspiration and ambition is rather thin. To aspire for one's betterment is valid and makes sense. However, vaulting ambition can often do more harm than good. This difference needs to be understood thoroughly by corporate executives—both young and seasoned. For whatever reason, ambition has long been prized and promoted by managers across the business spectrum. It is viewed as the ladder to success. But executives are rarely advised to match their high ambition and stretch goals with their capabilities. The mismatch between the two often results in disillusionment for the executive as well as the company. Unrealistic as they are, puffed-up goals often go for a six.

Management pundits have for quite some time been working on and writing about the perils of high ambition. Ambitious goals have long been used as a motivational tool for managers. Most companies try to nurture the ambition instinct in their managers as a matter of policy. Working in a pro-ambition environment, many imbibe this trait on their own. Ill-researched self-help books particularly, also propel younger managers towards the path of ambition.

The strangest fact is that no proven research exists establishing a causal relationship between ambitious goal-setting and its successful attainment. On the contrary, research findings of four top business schools quoted by the *HBR* show that in many cases, goals do more harm than good to companies and individuals using them. According to the findings, 'The researchers identified "bad side effects" produced by goal-setting programmes, including a rise in unethical behaviour, a narrow focus, distorted risks, the corrosion of organizational culture and reduced intrinsic motivation.'

According to recent neuroscience research, in the case of goal-setting the brain works in a protective way, resistant to change. Management expert and author Ray Williams points out that any goals that require substantial behavioural change, or thinking-pattern change, will automatically be resisted. When fear of failure creeps into the mind of the goal setter, it becomes a 'de-motivator', setting off a desire to return to known, comfortable behaviour and thought patterns.

Goal-setting often brings to the fore the mismatch between ambitious objectives and the manager's competencies. Whenever we desire things we don't have, we set our brain's nervous system to produce negative emotions. Williams elaborates, 'Highly aspirational goals require us to develop new competencies, some of which may be beyond current capabilities. As we develop these competencies, we are likely to experience failures, which then become de-motivational. If the goal is not attained, we often engage in thinking we are failures, not good enough, not smart enough, not beautiful enough, not worthy of success. Goal setting also sets up an either-or polarity of success. The only true measure can either be 100 per cent attainment or perfection, or 99 per cent and less, which is failure. That can leave us excessively focusing on the missing or incomplete part of our efforts, while ignoring the successful parts. It also doesn't take into account random forces of chance.'

I have come across numerous examples of young and senior managers who have been driven by high ambition to venture into uncharted territories. There is nothing basically wrong in aspiring to work in new business domains. In fact, those with their eyes set on CXO positions are expected to have adequate exposure to all major functions in business. The CXO needs to be an all-round professional. Yet at the same time, the aspiring manager should honestly evaluate his existing competencies. Nothing can match scrupulous self-evaluation. After all, you know yourself best! But how many managers really assess themselves without bias before choosing new goals. I recall a highly competent chartered accountant who was efficiently heading the finance department of a business group. But he had the CXO slot as his goal for long and ultimately managed to convince the board to designate him as chief operating officer (COO). With the new designation came new responsibilities and the new COO found himself not up to the mark. After a few tumultuous months, he had to return to the finance function and ultimately seek employment elsewhere. Both the company and the employee suffered.

Many a time, young managers pull strings to wangle their dream position. This is almost a practice in our part of the world. Company bosses are flooded with recommendations from politicos, bureaucrats, etc. to push their favourites up the ladder. Little do they realize that those recommended are hardly qualified and experienced for the new position. In fact, had they been good enough, they would have been automatically promoted. The private sector still honours merit. In fact, it survives and grows because of its star managers. Those who manage to move up on the basis of recommendation and pressure should remember that they will last only till their patrons remain in power. But they damage the organization and their own prospects as well till they manage to stick to their positions. Bereft of merit, they find no takers once they lose their office. There is no substitute for merit.

Goal-driven youngsters also try to enter and rise in companies on the basis of 'fancy' degrees and diplomas from the plethora of educational shops which masquerade as universities abroad. Many manage to 'buy' qualifications from established foreign universities. Even USA's prestigious Ivy League institutions welcome hefty endowments. But will such qualifications make Richie Rich bright overnight? Will they prove to be an asset for the companies they serve? No wonder this route is usually adopted by kith and kin of company owners and chiefs.

So if companies have to grow, then their goal should be to employ the really meritorious. And it is not difficult to locate the brilliant; they shine. The other goal should be to provide them all-round training. Polishing a diamond makes it brighter. This type of goal-setting is more than welcome. It is the call of the day.

Never Too Late To Learn

June 2019

Mentoring has been an integral part of learning in the Orient for ages. Whether it be the scriptures, governance (raj dharma), the art of war, performing arts like music and dance, or principles of business and commerce, devoted pupils have attained knowledge of diverse subjects at the feet of great masters. The one-to-one guru-shishya parampara (teacher-student tradition) has been and, to some extent, still continues to be the edifice of our educational psyche and heritage.

The business education system has undergone a paradigm change since the time the guru-shishya system reigned supreme. One-to-one teaching is no longer feasible in these times, at least in the initial stages like graduation and post-graduation. But strangely enough, it is the West which has kept the East's ancient educational pattern alive. By laying emphasis on personalized tutorials, universities like Oxford, Cambridge and Edinburgh in the United Kingdom, Harvard, Yale, MIT and other Ivy League institutions in the United States, several equally prestigious varsities in the non-English-speaking countries have maintained the close relationship between the teacher and the taught. Students are expected to sweat no less than their professors by regularly interacting with them individually and then presenting interpretative, innovative and original writings on their respective subjects. The transfer of knowledge, therefore, is more spontaneous and seamless.

Also the widely prevalent Asian practice of learning by rote and regurgitating the same in the exam hall has no place in the above varsities. No wonder world-class and practically applicable research emanates from such institutions. Patents developed by them are registered and adopted or bought by business houses. Ironically, the practice of debating and querying (shastrarth) has virtually vanished from the original land of the guru-shishya tradition.

This age-old system has gained currency in the corporate world now and is popularly understood as mentoring. In this learning relationship there is no discrimination of age, position or gender. Though the mentor is usually senior in age and experience than the protégé, it can be the other way round too and is termed as reverse mentoring. Many senior executives need to learn about the latest office technology, social media, computers, etc. Here it is worthwhile to seek the help of a tech-savvy young executive from within or outside the organization. That is reverse mentoring.

So what is a mentor? He/She is one before whom you do not feel the need to pretend or sport a mask. You have to be your true self so that the mentor can gauge your weaknesses and strengths properly and enable you to be a better professional by the time the mentoring ends. But mentoring by just one person is not the be all and end all of learning. After all, one needs to develop expertise in several domains during one's career. Hence you may need several mentors to attain your full potential.

History is replete with examples of mentors helping their protégés achieve memorable successes. Chanakya was instrumental in the rise of Chandragupta Maurya as emperor and was chief adviser to Chandragupta and his son Bindusara. Alexander would not have achieved greatness but for his tutor Aristotle.

Moving to the modern business era, Apple co-founder, the late Steve Jobs, was a mentor to Facebook co-founder Mark Zuckerberg. On Jobs' demise in 2011, Zuckerberg posted on his Facebook page, 'Steve, thank you for being a mentor and a friend. Thanks for showing that what you build can change the world. I will miss you.'

PepsiCo's former CEO Indra Nooyi observed, 'If I hadn't had mentors, I wouldn't be here today. I'm a product of great mentoring, great coaching...coaches or mentors are very important.' It's mentoring that helped her break the business glass ceiling and reach the top. Nooyi has figured in Forbes' list of 100 most powerful persons in the world.

It is evident that mentoring can do wonders both for the individual and the organization. Many companies see great benefit in institutionalizing the mentoring process. For example, accounting giant Deloitte has been a regular practitioner of mentoring; the objective is to ensure that the leadership pipeline is never vacant. Its Emerging Leaders Development Program keeps on preparing executives with leadership potential through mentoring.

Deloitte's website informs that each program participant is assigned a partner, principal, or director-sponsor who commits to at least two years to help their protégés drive their own careers by helping them understand how to steer their organization. When Deloitte's bright stars find the company so concerned about the blossoming of their talent they feel like staying on with the organization. Employee engagement and retention increases and attrition decreases. This is a big advantage as retaining top-notch managers is a real challenge for companies.

Shedding light on Intel's mentoring process, management thinker Vidya Hattangadi comments, 'Intel takes a slightly different approach to many other Fortune 500 companies. Rather than focus on hierarchy (connecting junior employees with senior employees), Intel focuses on specific knowledge transfer and domain skills that are in demand in present times.

'This philosophy is practised by the fact that everyone has something to learn—and everyone has something to teach. Intel's mentoring programme is less formal and more entrenched in the culture, resulting in more organic connections. The strength of Intel's mentoring programme lies in its momentum; rather than a coordinator managing and overseeing the programme like a hawk, employees take much of the process into their hands and take charge of their own learning.'

As I had mentioned in the beginning, reverse mentoring is prevalent more in multi-generational workplaces, whose numbers are growing. Here, the mentoring process involves matching senior executives with millennials to exchange fresh perspectives and encounter new ways of thinking about issues like technology, social media and current trends. Somehow many people tend to believe that mentoring should be within the company. But it has been found that executives can learn more from mentors who represent an external business culture and offer novel insights.

A former football coach, Bill Campbell mentored and changed the ways of a host of Silicon Valley's mighty CEOs. The *Investor's Business Daily* described the famous mentor thus: 'As a coach, Bill Campbell was willing to go to any lengths to change an executive's bad behaviour—up to and including telling his/her mom.' His protégés included the biggest names in technology like Steve Jobs, Jeff Bezos, Larry Page and Eric Schmidt. He was known for his plain-speak.

True mentoring is also gender-neutral. The assumption that female protégés prefer female mentors to learn growing and rising in male-dominated spheres is also without empirical basis. On the contrary, it has been found that female managers tend to learn better from male mentors, especially in science, technology, engineering and mathematics.

Given this backdrop, institutionalized mentoring can serve as a cost-effective tool for enhancing management standards in Nepal. It may be difficult for most companies to hire foreign mentors. But there is no dearth of knowledgeable and highly experienced Nepali promoters, entrepreneurs and top corporate executives. They need to take the initiative to share their treasure trove of skills to build a new generation of proficient management professionals.

Mentoring is a two-way traffic. Those who share knowledge will also get a lot in return in terms of employee loyalty, insight into human resource behaviour, and also the innovative spirit which the youth have in abundance.

Management Lessons From
Mumbai's Dabbawalas

July 2019

Ordinary beings can often do extraordinary things and set an example for management bosses and dons without holding fancy qualifications or undertaking expensive business training programmes. I am going to talk about a group of people, many of them semi-literate, who have set global benchmarks in the service industry. They consider their customer to be God. With such customer-centricity, they can only excel.

I am talking about the dabbawalas (tiffin service operators) of Mumbai whose virtually flawless service has become a case study in top B-schools like Harvard. Unlike popular perception, dabbawalas are not caterers. In ultra-busy Mumbai, the world's fourth most populous city, it is they who keep thousands of office-goers well fed daily.

Commuting in congested Mumbai is an ordeal. Local trains form the lifeline of local transport. But they stop for just 60 seconds at major stations and for 40 seconds at smaller ones. The typical Mumbaikar has to leave home for office by 7–7.30 a.m., reach the nearest local railway station and then fight his way into a jam-packed train compartment. The commuter often misses a train or two before being able to squeeze his way into one.

This being the routine, the commuter is not able to carry fresh food from home so early in the morning. Moreover, it is almost impossible for him/her to carry a tiffin box in an overcrowded compartment. Thus arises the need for someone to pick up the tiffin with fresh warm food from the office-goer's home and deliver it to his/her office by lunchtime. The empty tiffin has to be returned to the customer's house by the evening. The dabbawalas provide this valuable service day in and day out enabling office-goers to get hygienic home food of their taste. Let me present some statistics to explain the process: Firstly, dabbawalas are not caterers. The steel or aluminium tiffin box and its food contents belong to the customer. In Mumbai, dabbawalas deliver your food from your home to your workplace before lunchtime. Once lunch is over, they deliver your empty tiffin container back to your home the same day. That means they make two deliveries a day.

The dabbawala system was started in Mumbai by Shri Mahadev Havaji Bachche in 1890 with about hundred men. As the business grew, a charitable body by the name of Nutan Mumbai Tiffin Box Suppliers Trust was registered in 1956. The trust turned commercial in 1968 under the registered name Mumbai Tiffin Box Suppliers Association. The association's current employee strength stands at 5,000. The average literacy rate of the employees is eighth grade. The number of tiffins/customers is two lakh (200,000). Thus, including the returns of the tiffin, four lakh service transactions happen every day. So the annual transactions reach a figure of 12 crore (4,00,000 x 25 days x 12 months = 120,000,000). Each employee covers 60–70 km daily. He usually carries 40 tiffin boxes weighing a total of 60–65 kg. The time taken for the entire exercise is eight to nine hours. But the morning's three hours—9 a.m. to 12 noon—are like wartime.

You would be surprised to learn that not once in their history of 129 years have the dabbawalas failed to deliver the tiffin in time even if the local trains are late or it is raining cats and dogs as it often does in Mumbai. Riots, public rallies and even terrorist attacks have not been able to delay the *dabba* daredevils. Such is their commitment to customer service. They may not have heard of Six Sigma but they are its best practitioners. No wonder, the error rate is one in 16 million transactions. That translates into a Six Sigma rating of 99.99999. The dabbawalas have been delivering tiffins for more than a century, yet it was not until August 2011 that they halted services by observing a one-day strike in support of Anna Hazare, the revered anti-corruption activist.

Each group of 30–40 dabbawalas has a group leader called a mukadam. He is usually the eldest in the group. Though this position does not get him even an extra rupee, it's a matter of honour and prestige. He and also the other group members keep the names, addresses and phone numbers of the customers in their minds. No computers or laptops for them. Their passion for their vocation makes them extra efficient and vigilant. The monthly fee charged by the dabbawalas is also very reasonable: INR 1000— 1500 depending upon the distance to be covered. Diwali bonus is one month's extra payment. But the service is not discontinued if the customer refuses to pay the bonus. The logic is simple. Why miss 12 months' salary for one month's bonus. This is how customers are retained. However, we all know that schools and school buses charge for the entire year though schools remain closed for holidays for months. But the dabbawalas believe in maintaining unbreakable ties with their customers so much so that they won't charge a customer for the period he goes to his native town or elsewhere, sometimes for months. That is how the dabbawala-customer relationship lasts for decades, almost till the customer retires from his job and stops going to office.

It is this work ethos and passion for service that has prompted management gurus and teachers from the world over to study the dabbawala tradition. Professor Stefan Thomke, the William Barclay

Harding Professor of Business Administration at Harvard Business School and a leading authority on the management of business experimentation and innovation, spent considerable time in Mumbai to understand and study the operation and inner working, best practices and processes of this cadre of 'professionals'. The professor has worked with many global companies on product, process and technology development. It is also not sheer coincidence that the dabbawalas attracted worldwide attention and visits by Prince Charles, British entrepreneur Richard Branson, and employees of Federal Express, a company renowned for its own mastery of logistics. The Prince had even invited them to his marriage with Camilla in the year 2005.

Coming back to the good professor's findings, let me provide a summary for the benefit of young business managers. 'The dabbawalas' success is proof that with the right system in place, ordinary workers can achieve extraordinary results,' Professor Thomke stated in his article in the *HBR*. 'The dabbawalas have an overall system whose basic pillars—organization, management, process, and culture—are perfectly aligned and mutually reinforcing. In the corporate world, it's uncommon for managers to strive for that kind of synergy. While most, if not all, pay attention to some of the pillars, only a minority address all four. Culture, for example, often gets short shrift: Too few managers seem to recognize that they should nurture their organizations as communities—not just because they care about employees but because doing so will maximize productivity and creativity and reduce risk.' Stating it in a nutshell the professor added, 'The takeaway: managers shouldn't think of themselves merely as leaders or supervisors; they also need to be architects who design and fine-tune systems that enable employees to perform at optimal levels.'

It would be worthwhile for managers to get in-depth information about the dabbawalas' four pillars of strength and excellence and emulate them in their respective businesses.

Self-management For the Young and Restless

August 2019

Managers get work done. Yes, that is a manager's job, his work, his test. But how does he do that? Through self-management, the cardinal principle for a manager from day one! But this is not an easy principle to practise. Getting work done by one's team and a large number of external shareholders can be quite challenging. Many young and mid-level managers have experienced this reality and rued why they did not focus on a vital competency like self-management in time. But it is never too late to begin the journey for betterment.

Only a manager who has mastered the art of managing himself/herself can marshal his/her inner resources to get work done by others. However, a mere high intelligence quotient (IQ) would not make you a great manager. The aspiration for success demands that the young manager be fully equipped to deal with his physical, mental, emotional, social and spiritual realms. He will be required to face challenges from any or all of these domains during his career.

Though help from seniors and mentors may be at hand, the young manager can shine in his company or industry only if he practises self-help. This is because only he can best understand his strengths and weaknesses. So it devolves upon him to improve his faculties. Self-management is all the more vital today as the world has become a global village. Thanks to incredible advances in technology, a manager often has to do business with persons he may have never met personally. Many of his team members may be located abroad. This situation demands special abilities to get work done remotely. Self-management needs perfect coordination between body and mind. Today's strenuous work pace demands both physical and mental fitness. While young managers have woken up to the need for physical fitness, they are largely clueless about ways to master the mind. How should they train the mind? Yoga is the answer.

In yoga, one should start with meditation. Sit alone in a quiet place daily and let thoughts enter and exit the mind. Gradually try to focus on one thought which could be your deity or pure formless consciousness. There are various ways of meditation. You can choose one of them or take the help of a yoga instructor. With time, you will find that your mind has become better at focusing on the issue of your choice. Such mental focus will make your responses to managerial challenges more stable and sturdy. You will also not feel fatigued after a day of intense work.

Your attitude towards work will determine your performance. Attitude forms the core of karma yoga philosophy. Nishkaam Karma is all about acting proactively and putting your best foot forward without calculating what you will get out of it. This is a call to abandon selfishness believing that all good actions will result only in good outcomes. Otherwise, you will be besieged by anxiety and spoil the quality of your karma. Maintaining such a cool attitude in both success and failure is what has been described as equanimity (samabhav) in the Bhagavad Gita—*samatvam yoga uchyate.*

Leadership coach and author Susan Ritchie has elaborated upon some realistic and practical measures for self-management. Here is a summary.

Humility has been the hallmark of great leaders and managers. So, don't let ego overrule your better sense. Do not brag about your accomplishments. Leadership is, after all, a mix of inspiring and motivating others.

It is natural to be less confident in the initial phase of one's career. Young managers should remember that their low confidence level can be very easily noticed by their discerning team which may consist of persons senior to them in age and experience. It would be worthwhile to get hold of a seasoned mentor who ensures that you keep reminding yourself of your strengths. This can be an ever ready morale booster. Even then be prepared for mistakes to happen; nobody is perfect. Build your support network—a confidant, a coach, a guide—who keeps inspiring you and helps you keep a balanced view of your strengths and successes. Sharpen your listening skills. Listening attentively to the person in front of you forms the better part of communication but is, unfortunately, the most underrated managerial tool. By listening properly you make the other person feel important. Your relationship gets stronger. So, listen, learn and succeed.

Remain emotionally cool. Losing your cool makes you look weak. Good managers are expected to be warm and strong, calm and in control.

The ability to prioritize your goals and actions is of paramount value. Do not get distracted by someone else's agenda or your to-do list may not reflect your objectives.

You are the best judge of your time. Therefore, devise appropriate systems and processes so that you utilize your time judiciously and optimally. Convey it to your team as well. Educate your team about how and when you will be available. You need not be available all the time!

Be careful about your focus as you switch over to new roles. One usually wants to continue with tasks one is good at. But as you climb the corporate ladder your roles will change too. Alter your focus accordingly. Be prepared to move out of your comfort zone. New roles and responsibilities demand extra effort. Getting acclimatized to the new environment can be tough and energy-sapping and stressful. You therefore need to maintain, rather, boost your energy levels. Take small breaks during the day to overcome the pressure and tedium of work. Equally significant is physical well-being. Proper nutrition, exercise and work-life balance will ensure regular high performance from you.

Self-care and self-management go hand in hand. Yes, you can do it yourself.

Economics, Economics and Economics

October 2019

Readers of 'Business Sutra', a regular column published in the *Business 360°* magazine, must have realized by now that the column is devoted largely to tools and techniques of management. Though aimed at young and upcoming business executives, the column offers something for all managers across the spectrum of age and domains. However, the current upheavals in the global economy demand that we focus on the relevance and significance of the study of economics for managers. If you think deeply enough, you will realize that whether it be manufacturing, trade, marketing, sales, distribution, finance, HRD or R&D—all are creatures of the economy. Yet economics does not find the pride of place in B-school curricula. What a pity!

For a manager or a corporate house to succeed it is imperative to keep a hawk's eye on the changing patterns of the economy. Economies go through ups and downs. They also display easily discernible cyclical patterns. All through this, we also witness birth and demise of concepts and products. Nothing lasts forever. Yet there is no dearth of instances when managers remained so engaged in the nitty-gritty of business operations that they lost sight of the bigger picture—the economy.

Changes in economies happen all too frequently now as the world has become globalized. A major economic development thousands of kilometres away can rock your boat here, so strong and dynamic are the current business linkages. We cannot wish this away and run an insular business sitting in our silos. The sooner young managers in Nepal internalize this reality the better.

No wonder corporate behemoths the world over employ top-notch economists to keep a tab over global, national and local economies. The idea is to get advance notice of the changes rumbling in the distance. There is no point waking up when the elephant is in the room. Once the jumbo appears you are left with little choice. It's the giant animal who will decide whether to trample you or pamper you. Once you are adequately informed, you, in consultation with the top management, calibrate your policies, strategies and tactics accordingly. The tools of management that you have been equipped with at the business school and in real life business interaction can then be used differently to tackle the changing scenario.

Why am I urging young managers to brush up their knowledge and understanding of economics as an academic discipline? Because this academic stream can enable you to identify and tackle practical problems in your business like a champion gladiator. You should be aware of the global economic slowdown which is sending shivers down the spine of governments, policymakers and even the common man. In fact, the common man is the most vulnerable when an economic meltdown occurs. Businesses too are battered but most of them have the resilience to rise again and live another day. Unfortunately, the common man does not enjoy this luxury and ends up ruined.

Let's find out how pervasive is the current economic slowdown and how it has pulled down demand, consumption and investment. This is not the forum to go down deeply into the 'why' and 'how' of the economic turmoil. (Suffice it to say that the US-China tariff war, US economic sanctions against Iran and the recent attack on Saudi oil facilities are some, only some, of the major reasons stoking fear of a potential global recession.) But understanding its fallout is certainly the need of the hour for young managers. How else will they be able to brace themselves against the looming crisis?

Let's begin with the state of affairs in the US. The annual economic growth rate of the world's number one superpower fell to 2.1 per cent in the second quarter, down from 3.1 per cent in the first three months of 2019. This was caused by a 5.2 per cent drop in exports on account of economic weakness in Europe and trade war with China and other countries. The trade war has taken a toll on manufacturing. According to the US Commerce Department, a drop in business investment and investments in commercial and residential real estate have also contributed to the economic deceleration. Randy Kroszner, a former governor on the Federal Reserve Board, said, 'Trade policy uncertainty weighs on companies. They have to think about "Do I invest now do I invest later?" '

European Central Bank President Mario Draghi is worried over the outlook getting "worse and worse" in the Eurozone. The European Commission's Business Climate Indicator has been in its worse dropping mode in the last six years. A recent Bank of France survey revealed that the country's manufacturing sector growth plunged to a six-year low in June because production in the auto sector, plastics and electronics slowed down. ArcelorMittal had to temporarily lay off 1,400 Italian workers for 13 weeks at its Taranto plant. Europe's largest economy, Germany, just about avoided a recession last year. Decline in exports amid concerns of a global slowdown was the cause. GDP fell by 0.1 per cent quarter on quarter. That takes down Germany's annual growth rate to a measly 0.4 per cent. Economic analyst Andrew Walker opined, 'This is the downside of being an exporting powerhouse. When the international economic environment clouds over, you get rained on... China is at the centre of trade storms and it's also an important export market for Germany. So trade held the economy back...'

The British Chambers of Commerce (BCC) has disclosed that Britain is set on a course for the most prolonged slump in 17 years because of the global economic slowdown and the US-China trade war. *The Guardian* reported, '...business spending was due to decline by 1.5 per cent in 2019 and 0.1 per cent the next year as companies put their investment plans on ice amid the global political turmoil.' BCC has warned that investment in the UK will fall for three years consecutively.

What about China, which is at the centre of the global crisis? Well, the slowdown in the world's number two economy registered in August its weakest industrial production in over 17 years. Retail sales and investment figures have fallen despite the government introducing several growth boosting measures since 2018. The tariff war with the US is bruising the dragon badly. Industrial output growth unexpectedly weakened to 4.4 per cent in August month on month. Reuters reports that China has let its currency weaken, not a very honourable response in business and economic circles.

Singapore, the darling of business observers, has been jolted by the US-China trade slugging. CNN Business is of the view that the island nation could be headed for a recession. It reported its weakest annual growth since 2009 when its economy shrunk by 0.6 per cent. The wealthy nation chopped its GDP growth forecast in 2019 to between 0 per cent and 1 per cent. The previous prediction expected the economy to grow by between 1.5 per cent and 2.5 per cent. Singapore relies heavily on exports and China is its biggest trading partner. We have seen how slow the Chinese economy is moving for well over a year.

All this is worrisome for Nepal. But far more alarming is the slowdown in neighbouring India, the world's sixth-largest economy and the third-largest consumer market. Let's not forget that Nepal's last fiscal year, which ended this mid-July, accounted for 64.6 per cent (Rs. 63 billion) of our exports and 64.7 per cent (Rs. 918 billion) of our imports with India. Over 90 per cent of our international trade goods pass through India. The NPR is also directly pegged with the INR.

Although with a projected GDP growth rate of 5 per cent India is ahead of the other big countries except China (projected GDP growth 6.2 per cent), any fall in India's economy in comparison to its past performance is bound to affect Nepal directly.

Are we ready to face the crunch? Have we even evaluated and estimated the crisis potential? This is what Nepal's government, its private sector and most importantly, our forward-looking and hard-working young managers need to focus on.

When the going gets tough, the tough should get going.

Business Dharma

January 2020

A very happy new year to managers young and old!

It is for over a year that 'Business Sutra' has been my platform for discussing the art and science of management with young managers and executives. Globalization of real politics and business has ushered in phenomenal changes in the domain of commerce, trade and economics. The changes continue to occur torrentially. Managers today feel compelled to remain on their toes and on top of the learning curve. Most new management concepts and practices have been emanating from the western world. Japan too has not lagged behind and has made its indelible mark, particularly in the manufacturing sector. The Chinese management style is also attracting the business world's attention.

The last few decades have witnessed growing knowledge synergy between business practitioners and management academics. This intermingling of ideas has given birth to business solutions which are more worthy of practice and implementation. But it is a pity that business corporations and managers in Nepal and many neighbouring countries still rely largely on imported knowledge. This approach carries several risks. Firstly, foreign knowledge is not rooted in our culture and social psyche. Often English words and phrases fail to perfectly convey all our ideas because of a cultural mismatch. It is, therefore, difficult to implement and replicate imported concepts successfully in our socio-business reality. One size does not fit all. Secondly, over-reliance on external ideas impedes the growth of indigenous thinking. We need to focus on our problem areas and come up with solutions which match our way of thinking and living. The success rate of such suggestions will be much higher. Blindly aping the Western way of business cannot help Nepal beyond a point. We need to go *swadeshi* to achieve our true potential and make our successes sustainable.

So what is the way out? Or should I say what could be the way out for Nepal? There are no readymade and customized solutions for the plethora of business enterprises in both the manufacturing and service sectors. What can Nepali businesses do to ensure congruity between the goals and beliefs of the companies and their employees, including managers? Harmony prevails and business grows when there is a healthy matching. However, in the Western system, we see employees being manipulated through compensation alone. It is believed that compensation is motivation enough. Extensive business research has shown that nothing can be further from the truth. We all are familiar with the old aphorism that man does not live by bread (read money/financial benefits) alone. The most loved and respected companies are not always the best paymasters. There is much more than money that keeps a man going beyond his best.

To bring companies and their managers on the same page one can always take recourse to our scriptures. The suggestion may appear orthodox or plain stupid to some ultra-modern managers. I will not fault them because for a very long time our youngsters have been made to believe that spiritual scriptures and day-to-day life do not go together. It is asserted that scriptures are meant only for the religious and pious folk in the evening of their lives. This is patently wrong.

Firstly, there is not much common between religion and spiritualism. One can follow the Hindu way of life without being religious in the conventional sense of the term. You need not believe in and pray to multiple deities. At the same time, you may do so if you so wish to. You can repose all faith in any deity of your choice even if you create one for yourself. There is no dearth of gram (village) or vandevtas (forest deities) and devis (goddesses) in Nepal and this part of the world. You will not lose your place in the Hindu social structure even if you do not believe in a god. Moreover, Hindu scriptures do not talk of a specific form of God.

The Hindu way of life is all about following *dharma* or the righteous way of caring for all without any distinction. As the Bhagavad Gita (the Celestial Song) tells us, a worldly person can very well pursue the four chief aims of life, namely, dharma, artha (wealth), kama (sensual desires) and moksha (liberation). People from diverse domains of life and society have followed the Bhagavad Gita's teachings for millennia. It is among the most popular spiritual guides cutting across religions, climes and countries. This is so because the Gita talks of universal love and welfare; it is non-sectarian. That being the case anyone can seek spiritual, moral and ethical sustenance from the Bhagavad Gita, the Vedas, Upanishads, and epics like the Ramayana and Mahabharata. Business managers, junior to senior, are no exception. In fact, the dilemma about right and wrong has become all the more acute in these globalized times. If businesses are sprouting, they are dying too in large numbers. Anxiety about job security has reached alarming levels. The human spirit is getting jolted by the vicissitudes of rocking business patterns. Social and family structures are crumbling. The western business model is not human enough to deal with the situation. It is marked by inequity and inequality.

In this hour of crisis, should we not retrieve our ancient value systems which have been the bedrock of Nepali society since times immemorial? I would like to reiterate my emphasis on our ethical and moral construct. We might have strayed from the right path. We need to get back to it. Simultaneously, we need to banish those regressive practices which have sneaked their way into the Hindu way of life and its deep spiritual foundations. Companies will thus rejuvenate not only themselves but the entire Nepali society. What could be the righteous path for managers in this scheme of things? What should be their duties to ensure order, harmony and growth in business and personal life? The scriptures deal in detail about duties like planning, organizing, staffing, coordinating and controlling organizations or states. Here is some knowledge distilled from the Bhagavad Gita

To follow the path of dharma, managers should embrace virtue as a part of life. By identifying himself with virtue, a manager will be able to keep himself away from personal considerations for short-term gains and selfish agendas. By acting selfishly without keeping other stakeholders in the loop, the manager becomes solely responsible for the results he reaps. Consultative process is always a better option and acts as a multiplier. Straying from the righteous course leads to self-destruction. The manager should accord precedence to organizational goals and align his targets with them. This creates a win-win situation and also engages the organizational strength in the manager's karma. Every manager knows that the outcome of his efforts is not in his hands. Despite the best of intentions his contribution can get affected by his own infirmities as well as other factors like competition, unethical adversaries, changes in business and market scenario, etc. Therefore, the best way is to focus on the process, details and monitoring of the action (karma) rather than the result. This is what we call Nishkaam Karma. A job well done is good enough for satisfaction. Even the best manager cannot claim a perfect strike rate.

By detaching himself from an uncertain outcome the smart manager gains clarity in decision-making. A manager ridden by anxiety about the result fumbles in his actions and may opt for irrational steps. A clear and steady mind is the manager's best associate. One can develop equanimity through the practise of yoga.

Kautilya's Arthashastra focused, among other things, on financial matters. Way back in the fourth century BC Kautilya or Chanakya described nyaya (justice) and dharma (ethics) as the fundamentals of governance. He stressed upon regular audit of public services. Significantly, he was all for task orientation rather than target orientation in auditing. The Mahabharata is a veritable treatise on leadership—a core area of modern management.

We have so much to imbibe from what we already own. Will we do that?

Listen To Feedback

February 2020

You get back what you feed in. In fact, you get back more than what you give. That is the magic of feedback in business management. So, if you are in any way linked to managing business, then you would certainly be aware of the all-round role and significance of feedback. Yet, there is lack of clarity about the concept. The general feeling is that feedback is all about a senior manager periodically evaluating his juniors' performance. This has given rise to the belief that it is only a bi-annual or annual practice.

From the textbook point of view, this perception is way off the mark. But practice-wise, it is quite on the mark. This is how feedback is generally used as an HR tool in our part of the world. And it would be worthwhile to dwell on this topic alone in this piece.

However, before I move further, let me clarify a few issues for our young managers. Feedback is an integral part of all managerial functions. It impacts all participants in business whether they are customers, clients, employees, suppliers, vendors, bankers, knowledge providers or any other stakeholders. Adherence to this approach will ensure that your company continues to excel on all fronts. How can an enterprise improve continuously without actively finding out what is wrong or lacking in different business functions? Effective and timely feedback, both positive and negative, is a vital ingredient of a successful performance management and goal setting programme. It drives human resource development.

Let's start with the easier system—*positive* feedback. Though easier to deliver, positive feedback is not provided as often as it should be. In our society, it is generally believed that praise may go to the employee's head and make him either more demanding or complacent. I have observed the majority of senior managers only pulling up and reprimanding their junior colleagues. That is their view of the feedback system. This is a fallacious notion which is injurious to relationships in the workplace. However, by turning negative feedback into constructive criticism managers can change the game altogether for the better. So, let's get down to understanding the art and science of constructive feedback.

A pat on the back can enormously boost an employee's morale and make him more productive. It also creates a nurturing and supportive culture in the organization. Feedback needs to be *timely*. It needs to be given soon after a specific behaviour or event. If you pull up an employee months after some bad behaviour or event, do not expect an effective outcome. In fact, the employee may not be able to even link your criticism to the real event after so long. Also, he may not recognize the severity of his folly because of the delay. He would be right to assume that had his error been so grave you would have taken up the issue with him immediately. The delay renders the feedback futile. The same holds true when the manager delays words of praise after a good deed or exceptional performance. Delayed appreciation loses its impact. Frequent but deserved acclaim adds to productivity.

While timeliness of applause is certainly essential, no less imperative is the *specificity* of the feedback. It is no good telling an employee that he is going downhill or, conversely, going great guns.

Full details of the good work done or the mistakes committed by the employee should be provided to him/her in a feedback. The senior manager will need to fully prepare to provide solid, actionable and credible comments. *Feedback based on empirical data* is always more effective. For example, a positive feedback for a young marketing executive could be in terms of the target-plus sales leads generated by his campaigns. A negative feedback for a production manager could be about a statistically significant fall in goods produced even as related circumstances remained unchanged. For example, say, 23 per cent fewer goods were produced in a given period of time despite the fact that availability of raw material, electricity, labour, etc. faced no shortage. This will make it easier for the appraisee to fathom the loss that his act of omission or commission has caused to the company. This is justified feedback as it rules out possible foul play or vendetta by the feedback provider.

Feedback is not for the sake of giving back. The objective is to make good performers do better and enable low performers to rectify mistakes, avoid repeating errors and become more accomplished. Therefore, the appraised employee should also be suggested *practical and doable measures to improve performance.*

While this constitutes the crux of the feedback mechanism, there are some smaller yet significant facts that reinforce the system. Feedback delivery should never be turned into a public circus. One has often seen senior managers hauling up their juniors in front of all. This amounts to deliberate insult. Not only does the junior executive get thoroughly demoralized and crestfallen, he also loses respect among his peers. This affects the department's functioning adversely. An open interaction should certainly happen but at a relatively secluded and private place in the office where both parties are not overheard.

Then, the *language and manner of feedback delivery* determines its efficacy. Too many negative phrases often lead to the appraisee shutting down his mind. A barrage of negatives like 'shouldn't', 'don't', 'wasn't', etc. unnerves the person at the receiving end so much so that he is unable to state his case. He is then unable to absorb what he is being told. The entire feedback exercise thus comes to nought. Mixing debilitating criticism with the opportunity to the receiver to give his views as well can take care of the above challenge. It is, therefore, best to have a judicious mix of negative and positive points in the dialogue. The feedback provider should never be on an embarrassing spree. Unfortunately, this does happen when superiors lose their objectivity.

Most of us would remember good teachers asking us frequently during the class period whether they had been able to make themselves understood. This would encourage even the shy students to clear their doubts. It is the same with feedback. Experienced managers do the same while interacting with both good and bad performers. This can make even the toughest talk a motivating and learning experience. Both the feedback giver and receiver emerge enriched from this HRD experience.

Feedback can often get cramped when too many issues are stuffed in a single interaction. The human mind has its limitations. Absorbing unexpected criticism on a plethora of issues in a go can be mentally debilitating for the person under the glare. That is why so much emphasis is laid on timely delivery of one's comments. When that happens spontaneously, the possibility of confrontational issues piling up gets mitigated. A to-the-point and limited feedback has a higher success rate.

Wishing you fruitful feedback sessions!

AI: Threat or Opportunity?

March 2020

Artificial intelligence (AI) and reality may appear contradictory but the fact is that AI is fast becoming the reigning reality of modern life. AI is no longer a mere buzzword. Its potential applications are visible all around us from gaming to expert medical diagnostic systems to speech recognition to machine learning to robotics to customer services to workload automation and predictive maintenance to effective data management and analytics, etc. Sounds magical? Simply put, AI is computer software that performs human-like activities including learning, planning and problem solving.

According to an AFP news report from Washington in the latter half of February, US researchers used AI to identify an antibiotic chemical which can kill several drug-resistant bacteria generally known as superbugs. 'The scientists at MIT and Harvard trained a machine learning algorithm to analyse chemical compounds capable of fighting infections using different mechanisms than those of existing drugs,' the report stated. The identified compound has been, interestingly, named 'halicin' after the fictional AI system from '2001: A Space Odyssey'. The scientists succeeded in their quest for a new drug through a machine learning model that enabled them to explore large chemical spaces which without AI is a prohibitively expensive process even for advanced countries and pharmaceutical giants. Without new drugs, it is feared, resistant infections would be able to claim 10 million lives a year by 2050.

The news brings hope and reassurance to mankind at a time when the deadly corona virus (COVID-19) is spreading its tentacles beyond China, the country of its origin. Horror and terror abound. There is no immediate treatment in sight. However, it is believed that AI will enable us to find a way out sooner than later. If and when that happens, it will create immense opportunities for medical and pharmaceutical organizations and people at large.

AI has helped us make unimaginable advancements in different domains of human life. Robots are already teaching and assisting humans in conducting classes for junior students in a highly interesting and absorbing manner. Robots are running machines in automobile companies. Cars are moving around without drivers. Thanks to AI solving humongous calculations in a jiffy, creating new scientific models has become much easier and faster. Repetitive work may no longer be forced upon us. AI will take care of that while humans will devote themselves to real value-adding tasks. This is changing the way we have been doing business for too long. The development will only gain vigour and momentum over time. Managers in Nepal need to gear themselves up for the world-altering change.

Let's listen to AI expert Deidre Paknad. He says, 'Compared to humans, AI is able to crunch numbers, identify patterns, and make faster data-driven decisions. With the ability to process large amounts of data and spit out trend directions and actionable advice, this application of artificial intelligence can be a vital tool for any manager looking for some quantitative support in his decision-making. In fact, computers can be so good that in financial services, 40 per cent of predicted layoffs in the industry will be in money management, as robo-advisors replace human fund managers.'

According to a *HBR* survey of project managers, 54 per cent of their time was spent tackling routine administrative chores. This neither adds value to business nor does it motivate top-class managers. They are always on the lookout for challenging assignments whose accomplishment gives them a sense of fulfilment. AI is an excellent tool for such aspiring high-flyers. AI can assist good managers in bolstering team spirit by giving timely feedback. AI can manage regular, even weekly feedbacks, to team members by using natural language processing and chatbots. Global surveys have highlighted employees' faith in 'more' feedback. They feel that feedback and the consequent coaching and mentoring lead to better performance. With timely fact-based feedback, course correction can be made as and when it is required. AI offers means and tools to managers to identify team members who need more attention and guidance. It helps managers to anticipate the coaching needs of their team members.

We often come across AI in the manufacturing sector. The machines are connected to a network that supplies large amounts of data which is just too much to be sorted out and managed by humans efficiently. Machine learning comes into play here recognizing patterns and anomalies in the data rapidly. The managers concerned are immediately informed of the disruption in patterns, and corrective measures are taken to make the machines run as required.

Far more useful than machine learning is the new concept of deep learning. The algorithms used in this case equip machines with the power of non-linear reasoning. We can see this in operation in self-driven cars whose sensors are able to gauge distance from other objects in nanoseconds. Fraud detection ability too is gradually making deep learning highly useful for businesses with growing availability of data.

The customer, we fully realize, is the king in today's highly competitive business scenario. We are aware of customer relationship management softwares like Salesforce and Zoho. But these need a high level of human intervention. Application of AI to these platforms can imbue them with the ability to auto-correct and self-update.

The best role that AI can play is protection of computer network defences. It can detect breaches in the defence system. No doubt there are cybersecurity experts but can a company afford to employ as many as warranted by the scale and complexity of computer networks? AI comes to the rescue here.

All this appears to be hunky-dory. But should a country like Nepal, which is majorly reliant on the old age economy, welcome AI with open arms? Our linkage with the knowledge-based economy is, at best, basic and tenuous. Education-wise, our people are equipped for basic jobs. On the other hand, AI seems to be an employment destroyer, particularly in the Nepali context. Nepal's business barons and managers need to seriously debate the issue. We may or may not adopt AI as willingly as many countries are doing but history shows that technology has a way of breaching barriers of forbidden lands. Moreover, we are already linked to a globalized world. External influences cannot be wished away. At best, we can induct AI in measured and calibrated doses. We need to understand enough of AI to be able to interact with the outside world. The advanced countries will not lag behind so that Nepal may catch up with them. Inequity has been the only permanent feature of humankind and it is set to increase. AI may only contribute to this horrid reality.

How to deal with this challenge? Thankfully, Nepal has a small population. We should change our national priorities to focus sharply on basic education and IT. We have seen that the world's best and most successful IT entrepreneurs were not college toppers. On the contrary, many of them were college dropouts. This is not to suggest that our youth should start disdaining higher education. What I am saying is that IT programming and coding skills require a burning zeal rather than certificates and degrees which are often not worth the paper they are printed on. Also, IT education and industry do not require big capital expenditure unlike education in other streams and the manufacturing sector.

The state, business and society need to create an enabling atmosphere and let a million flowers bloom.

Leveraging Social Media

June 2020

COVID-19 continues its tantrums. Protective lockdown is in force. We sit huddled in our homes, wary and scared. Normal communication is conspicuous by its absence. Social media has replaced it with new meaning.

With so much time at hand, I manage to comb through social media platforms rather earnestly. What have I discovered? Everyone is suffering tremendous pain and believes that someone else is responsible for the torment. Therefore, there is extraordinary venting of spleen. Among those being blamed for the misery are the people at the top, beginning from heads of states to politicos to government administration bosses to captains of industry to those running any organization which has anything to do with the public.

These days, the higher you are in the government, political or social pecking order, the greater is the probability of you being trolled to death in social media. Blame is the name of the game we are seemingly surviving by. But which sane creature would spend all his time and energy haranguing others for his misery instead of devising ways to make this protective imprisonment or, shall we say, preventive detention shorter and more bearable?

It is appalling to find social media so utterly bereft of concrete suggestions to fight the situation unleashed by the deadly virus at various levels. On the contrary, we are busy concocting conspiracy theories around COVID-19, creating fresh causes to squabble over by the minute.

Leaving apart God, who is supposedly beyond reproach, why is it that we only look upwards for succour and guidance? We will swear at the prime minister, the managing director, the vice chancellor, the police chief, the medical superintendent et al., and yet expect only them to resolve our problems. Such venomously ironical behaviour is perhaps the fallout of a long-practised paternalistic system. All this might have begun with a benign ruler taking care of his people like a benevolent father. But things change with time. One is not sure how and when the ruler became the all-powerful state and the people turned first into subjects and then into serfs. The business of thinking and making decisions became the state's prerogative. This made it one job less for the common man, till it started hurting.

By the time people woke up, it was too late, and like Rip Van Winkle, they found themselves in a new world. Now, they find it too hard to think on their own in real life. They are constrained to accept intellectual handouts from people above. But nothing comes for free. The benefactor doles away only what might fetch him good returns. This is the story of each and every aspect of life. In business too, those who dare to dream and have the guts to share their ideas rise to become leaders. Obedient and loyal executives remain followers. Have you ever wondered why most promoters prefer lapdogs? Because there is scant space at the top.

But the real leader knows no stopping. He quickly learns to marshal the infinite capability of his mind and air his thoughts even at the risk of being ridiculed. He suggests solutions and explanations. He is not into trading barbs; he is into sharing knowledge and ideas.

This takes him and his trade to new heights. He becomes the go-to guy when crisis strikes.

You too can seek and bring out the leader hidden inside you. Raise the bar for yourself. Search for obstacles proactively. Activate your neurons to discover solutions not excuses. You will soon find yourself changing into a sought-after leader.

COVID-19 Leadership Crisis

July 2020

Calamities can bring out both the best and the worst in leaders. The real test of leaders takes place when things turn tough. Those with real mettle do themselves and their people proud. They save nations.

The impact of COVID-19 on humankind has been unprecedented in intensity and magnitude. In its hitherto unending sweep, the virus pandemic is devouring lives, economies and businesses around the planet, cutting across communities, faiths, castes and creeds without discrimination. COVID-19 has been a great equalizer in that sense, killing rich and poor alike. The mightiest and richest of nations have been humbled by a microbe whose true nature and structure has defied the best scientific minds. And the anti-COVID-19 vaccine still remains a creature of human hope. The reality resides somewhere on the distant horizon. However scary and sordid the scenario may be, the virus has done well to shake off some of man's arrogance. Also, COVID-19 has put humankind in its place by reminding it that it is of its own making. So the suffering too will be borne by mankind. For too long have we been playing with Nature. Retribution direct and real has taken its toll so ruthlessly the first time in living memory.

Let's move to the more practical and pragmatic facet of the issue at hand. The idea is to analyse how political leadership can wreak havoc on all sections of its country or society because of its ideological predilections or sheer foolhardiness of a self-proclaimed charismatic leader.

Let's move to scenic Italy where most unseemly developments crushed the country's medical infrastructure and people's spirit. It needs to be noted that Italy is among the well-endowed countries of Western Europe. So far, its population of just over 60 million people was being ably serviced by one of the best healthcare systems in the region. Though the rate of infection is petering out in Italy in the first week of July with 34,854 scalps under its belt, the total infected cases thus far stand at 241,419. Of those currently infected (14,500 persons), 71 per cent are in a critical state. Indeed, these are disheartening numbers for a developed country!

To understand the Italian enigma, please incorporate another figure in the analysis. The number of Chinese living in Italy is approximately 310,000. The high number is explained by the recent spurt of Chinese investment in Italy: 29 deals worth $2.8 billion. Italy had been lagging behind other European Union (EU) countries vis-à-vis Chinese investment. But Italian trade zones and ports were soon open for China. Gratified by Beijing's largesse Italy chose to be in March 2019 the EU's only country to join China's much tom-tommed Belt and Road Initiative. Chinese tourists flocked to Italy. Following Covid's outbreak in China's Wuhan city, Italy suspended flights to China on 1 January 2020. But when China frowned upon the move, the Italian President Sergio Mattarello whimpered on 2 February that his country stood by China. Florence's Mayor Dario Nardella went to ridiculous lengths by urging the citizens to hug Chinese tourists and visitors in a show of solidarity. They did and COVID-19 caught Italy by the neck. Economic indebtedness to China cost Italy thousands of lives and its reputation too.

The COVID-19 crisis was also not well managed in Brazil. Stats first. Population: just over 21 crore; Deaths: 64,365; Cases: 1,578,376; Currently infected: 535,396 of which 2 per cent are in critical condition. Horrifying figures! A far-right fan of US President Donald Trump, the South American country's President Jair Messias Bolsonaro loved to describe COVID-19 as 'a little cold'. Voluntary quarantine seemed good enough to him. He blabbered on about miracle drugs even as thousands of his countrymen perished, medical infrastructure broke down, businesses fell apart and protesters rioted in the streets.

Similar erratic and arrogant behaviour has been often displayed by captains of industry. We have witnessed business behemoths simply vanishing from the world of commerce. The scope for destruction is enormous. Like civil society, young managers too have the responsibility to abide by ethics to contain unbridled autocracy within their corporations. Nobody is beyond the rule of law and corporate governance.

Yelling Bosses: Good or Bad?

August 2020

COVID-19 has created a new world; a nervy world. The death toll is rising. Health infrastructure is crumbling even in the most advanced and affluent countries. Global economy is in shambles. Jobs are being lost. Salary cuts have become the norm. Lockdowns have made people jittery and nervous. The future looks bleak. The pandemic's impact will be felt for years. Anti-COVID-19 vaccines seem to be the only silver lining beyond the dense clouds. But these are yet only being heard of, not seen.

In the business world, a very large number of managers and employees have been forced to work from home. Those who dare to go to office are being viewed as soldiers, not business executives.

The most vulnerable are the top managers who are responsible for delivering glowing results, quarter after quarter. They are at their nerves' end. Yelling and shouting at juniors has increased. Loudly reprimanding one's juniors and mentees has been part of the game forever, and not just in business. The best athletes and sportsmen rose to the top thanks to some of the harshest and foul-mouthed coaches. Yet, champions continue to consider such coaches no less than gods. In the armed forces too, non-commissioned sergeants have been known to train cadet officers into men of steel through methods not suitably suave and sophisticated. Their booming orders laced with unique abuses during parades, runs and battle drills are remembered with humour and respect even when officers become generals. The basics of real war and survival training imparted by the no-nonsense sergeants enabled many officers to return alive from the fiercest of battles with honour and glory.

Some of the younger managers may be feeling that I am building a case for regular and public scolding by their seniors. Certainly not! Even an entry-level manager has the sense to distinguish between malicious yelling and purposeful guidance by seniors even if done loudly and bluntly. You can easily find out whether the boss is shouting at you to give vent to his own frustration or to transfer the blame on to you for his own mistakes or, worse still, because he is inefficient and incompetent and has no solutions for your meaningful queries and doubts. Many a time, the knowledge and dedication of his young teammates intimidate an old-timer. Unable to keep pace with them, the senior tries to run them down by insulting them publicly or by carrying tales about them to higher-ups. The senior's insecurity makes life miserable for youngsters who start looking for companies with a better work culture. Ultimately, the company loses.

It is slightly difficult to recognize seniors who remain reserved, who set a gruelling regimen for you, give daunting assignments and give a pat on the back only when you perform outstandingly. They are frugal with laudatory words but you will really feel motivated when they smile at you. You will realize that you have earned the praise, have learnt new facts and have acquired new skills. You feel you are getting equipped for the fast track. Therefore, it does not matter if the senior has been rather gruff or not too amiable.

It is worth listening to author and management researcher Michael Schrage who stated in the *HBR*, 'To be sure, yelling does not make a better leader or manager. However, the notion that raising one's voice represents managerial weakness or a failure of leadership seems to be prima facie nonsense. The empirical fact pattern suggests that in a variety of creative and intensely competitive talent-rich disciplines around the world, the most successful leaders actually have yelling as both a core competence and brand attribute.' Schrage named Jack Welch, Bill Gates, Jeff Bezos, Steve Jobs etc. in support of his premise.

Having lent a perspective to yelling by bosses, let me caution you that you cannot wish obnoxious bosses away. They have been there and will continue to exist. How to deal with such overbearing creatures is an art in itself. We shall discuss that next.

Overbearing Bosses

September 2020

Dear readers, I had talked about yelling bosses earlier. The aim was to explain that most bosses and mentors do not scream their heads off just because they relish scaring young executives and managers. However, the fact remains that a small percentage of corporate biggies do deal with their juniors in a monstrous manner. Driven to the end of their tether, exasperated juniors are often forced to react in a fashion that damages their careers grievously. Such confrontations are best avoided.

What is the way out?

The first step in this direction involves winning the trust of your reporting manager. This is most relevant in corona times when several managers are working from home and any means of direct communication is disrupted. Your senior manager, who is responsible for producing predetermined results is working virtually in the dark. Used to interacting with his team in person, he may be confronted with a trust crisis during these days. He has no easy means to find out whether you are really working at home or taking cookery lessons or mending domestic electric gadgets. The situation makes the boss nervy. He feels he is no longer in control of things. Hence the occasional outbursts during telephonic interactions.

There are honest ways to avoid confrontations. Ensure that you are indeed working from home. You need to be organized. Whatever data can be procured in such circumstances should be at hand. This will make tele-calls or video calls more effective and fruitful. Figures, graphs and excel sheets should be kept ready to be displayed or transmitted to the boss on demand. Occasional calls and requests to the boss for doubt clearance and guidance enhances his trust in you. You both feel engaged in the same mission. Chances of spats get reduced. Mutual confidence grows.

Another way for a healthy relationship with the boss is proactive communication. Remember that the boss has the entire team reporting to him. You can make his life easier by e-mailing him your day's to-do or priority list first thing in the morning. Do mention pending goals and how you propose to catch up. A smart manager is expected to suggest possible solutions as well. Flooding the boss only with a laundry list of obstacles and problems is not going to take you too far. Despite being young and raw you are expected to be a thinking manager. This is the kind of communication needed at all times and especially so during extraordinary crises like the COVID-19 pandemic.

Despite your best efforts you may find that the boss continues to be overbearing, intrusive and domineering. It is time now to seek a direct one-on-one interaction with him, in person or electronically according to the situation. You should explain to the boss your way of working, your hits and misses, and your improvement plan. Do seek his specific, empirical and categorical views on what he considers a lackadaisical performance by you. Analyse the senior's critique. It is likely that he may be correct on certain points. You may have overlooked some of your shortcomings. It is also possible that part of your work style and personal goals may not be in alignment with the company's work culture and vision. Consider such a revelation a golden opportunity for course correction.

These are some of the right ways to mend ties with overbearing bosses. But getting a good boss is a matter of luck as well. Weak bosses will continue to micro-manage, yell and shout at you even if they come across one thing wrong among the hundred tasks you have done well, and never give credit for good work but on the contrary steal your bright ideas to move up the corporate ladder. Being nasty is the weak manager's defence mechanism. He tries to browbeat his juniors because he has no answers and solutions to their queries and challenges.

It is likely that you will fall prey to such bosses in companies or industries plagued by poor work cultures. You may, therefore, need to seek fresh pastures. Do that with a happy heart because the moribund companies you are leaving are doomed. Weak managers can take their companies in one direction only—down.

Head for the highway, bright ones! It will take you places.

The Reality of Job Loss and Salary Cuts

October 2020

Daring young managers with one bitter truth is better than ensnaring them with a thousand sweet lies. Yes, it needs to be openly admitted that redundancy or job loss and salary cuts are fast becoming a norm in the corporate world as COVID-19 continues to upset economies, companies and livelihoods across the globe. Nepal is no exception.

The country is suffering across sectors. Uncertainty, not hope, is the reigning sentiment. Tomorrow is another day. In this bleak scenario, young managers are most likely to be torn by anxiety. Many of them have lost jobs. Salary cuts have become common. With consumption drying up, businesses are drying up. Capital expenditure and growth have been reduced to pipe dreams. Survival seems to have become a universal goal. Though not of this scale, downturns have been a part of corporate life for as long as one remembers. Recessions, market crashes, natural cataclysms, wars and social strife have tested the grit and resilience of the business world time and again. It's time for managers and executives to rise to the occasion and live to fight another day.

Don't feel guilty about job loss or salary cuts. You are just one of the millions hit across continents. And like them, you are out of employment not because you are incompetent or inefficient. The COVID-19 crisis is one of its kind in human history. You are an innocent victim as economies are shrinking, countries are witnessing bleeding cuts in their GDPs, companies are adopting drastic measures to remain alive and the informal sector is falling apart. You can never be and will never be held responsible for your career predicament. So abandon anger, resentment and frustration and keeping your chin up, seek new and innovative ways of making a living.

First of all, take stock of your resources. How much money do you have in cash or in the bank? Make a reasonably tight budget for the next six months. You will be amazed to find how many expenses you can do without. Now get ready for job hunting. As I have already stated, you have no reason to be ashamed of being jobless. In fact, this is the time to spread the word in your network and outside.

As you will be approaching a diverse set of potential employers be ready to customize your résumé as per their requirements. One size does not fit all. Most young managers possess more than one skill set. Showcase relevant skills to each employer you approach. You should be mentally prepared to take up work which may not exactly match your previous experience or remuneration. Young managers are at an advantage in this respect as they are exposed to different roles in the initial phase of their work life. Only senior managers get identified with specific specializations and find it difficult to get equivalent jobs elsewhere. Comparatively, young executives have a vast playfield.

Remember that COVID-19 has compelled businesses to create and adopt unique ways of working. Working from home is not exactly new but has now gained currency in view of the infectious pandemic. Work does not always mean a full-fledged job. So why not offer your skills, say, accounting, digital marketing or HR functions, namely, payroll management, to more than one non-competing company on a part-time basis. In these uncertain times, it seems better to have more than one source of income. Many companies are now desisting from increasing permanent employees on their rolls for obvious reasons. They are preferring consultants for fixed amounts. Medium-size enterprises would like to avail the services and skills of managers with a business background, but for reasonable fees.

Pandemic-hit executives should try to ensure continuity in work as suggested above. Never sit idle if you have lost your job. There are many online courses for learning contemporary skills. You might as well start offering online advice to medium and small businesses or engage in result-linked projects. This work style may seem a little uncertain and dicey. But the days of certainty are gone and one needs to adapt to the changes. The sooner the business world learns it the better.

Be the Change You Want To See

November 2020

All are wondering what the world would be like once COVID-19 is controlled. Many feel it will be a different scenario altogether.

The corporate world is expecting a different work culture to emerge once things return to normal. In fact, we are already witnessing unprecedented changes in our life and work styles.

We are getting used to being confined to our homes following protective lockdowns. Work-from-home is becoming a reality with long-term socio-economic implications. While its economic impact is much talked of, the social impact has not drawn adequate attention. Though it is a separate issue in itself, I feel work-from-home may boost women's emancipation across societies. Digitization will make work and family life easier for both genders.

Focusing on the corporate world, one finds that medical and pharma enterprises have already adopted major changes in work systems in the global fight against the COVID-19 pandemic. See how pharma companies have abandoned deeply entrenched and proven protocols in their quest for a safe and effective vaccine against the deadly virus. The time span for developing a vaccine, which usually runs into years, is being compressed in view of the virus's inter-continental spread and lethality. Inter-country and inter-company collaborations are driving the vaccine search. The private and public sectors have joined hands. All this entails tremendous adjustments to diverse work cultures. Innovation and agility have become the keywords in this global endeavour whose history has yet to be chronicled.

However, it is becoming increasingly clear that the worst of times bring out the best in us. Faced with an existential crisis, people or companies perform miracles. The keen competition between different COVID-19 vaccine candidates proves the point. Scientists, pharma companies and countries are rapidly devising new ways to create an elixir against the deadliest viral contagion in living memory without compromising on safety and efficacy. It is apparent that new work systems are being evolved, tested and verified. This is a rocket-velocity change in work culture happening before our eyes.

It is, therefore, apparent that success on the vaccine front will only propel enterprises to make changes in their established ways much faster than before to introduce newer and better products and services. This will be a new world needing enterprising, agile, innovative and nimble-footed managements, executives, experts and other employees. Mere walking won't do. Skateboarding will become the new mode of mobility. Are our managers and young executives readying themselves for the times to come?

Is this sounding very daunting to young executives? Well, it should not. Change in work culture has been as old as business itself. The difference now is that it is becoming regular and faster. It has been noted that companies and managers who embraced change proactively remain ahead on the learning and growth curve, whereas those who opted for change when compelled by dipping business fortunes either fell by the wayside or simply languished. The new era will have place only for executives who are agile, nimble-footed, adjustable and innovative.

Let me bring to your attention a major exercise on work culture change in Dr G.K. Reddy's pharma MNC as reported in the *HBR* in June 2017. The company had, at that point of time, seven distinct units working in 27 countries with over 20,000 employees. Each unit had its own work culture. There were too many procedures and too much decision-making across the behemoth which was becoming a formidable challenge. After much deliberation the top management at Dr Reddy's decided that all its operations and employees needed to be nimble, innovative and patient-centred. To align and galvanize the company's manpower around this target the leadership came up with an inspiring purpose: 'Good health can't wait'. However, before announcing the purpose, small and modest projects were launched across channels to highlight agility, innovation and customer-centricity. The work involved many activities, from product packaging to creation of an internal data platform for employees to be proactive and agile when dealing with customer requests. After all, nothing can match successes and wins, even though small, to inspire and attract employees who are not easily impressed by mere slogans, however well thought out. Living examples carry a lot of weight. Therefore, even small successes need to be celebrated to establish the credibility and effectiveness of the real purpose of a project.

So all were asked how they could contribute to the guiding principle 'Good health can't wait'. One of the scientists reported how he had been able to develop a product within 15 days. This was amazing considering that procurement of raw material itself for creating a new product used to take months. The scientist was candid enough to disclose that he could achieve such a milestone only by ignoring long established procedures and using innovative practices.

It is a fact that companies often continue with old systems and procedures which have lost relevance.

Real change in work culture happens when employees start asking themselves 'why do we exist' beyond personal gains. And this did happen at Dr Reddy's through an elaborate change in work culture. Today, the company continues to prosper as do the employees.

To use a Gandhian phrase in this case, young executives need to be the change they want to see in their companies.

One and One Can Make Eleven

December 2020

Fear, like the wind, is invisible. It knows no boundaries. Therefore, its effect can be felt far and wide. COVID-19 is today the world's most globalized 'sentiment'. Fright, anxiety, uncertainty, confusion, erosion of faith and loss of trust are its most common symptoms. No domain of human life has been spared this dreaded syndrome.

In keeping with the basic theme of 'Business Sutra', I will be focusing on business and its practitioners. The travails being faced by young managers are bothering me the most. Having seen far fewer springs than old business hands, youngsters seem to be at their wits' end. But this is anything but their criticism. Hardly had they started their careers than they have been hit by the planet's worst crisis.

In times of adversity, the young usually look up to their elders, seniors, mentors and governments. That is the way the world functions. That is the way we have been brought up. Long-term guidance and support by the older generation is a given, more so in Nepal and neighbouring countries with strong family values. This culture covers our business sector too. Relationships matter a lot. The business owner is seen as a father or mother figure. And parents and their progeny cannot sever ties as clinically as is the practice in the West. Job cuts, salary reduction, business closures and other worse consequences of the rampant COVID-19 virus are, therefore, all the more painfully felt in Nepal. COVID-19 is claiming lives as the feeble public health infrastructure is crumbling because of the dreaded disease's deadly blow. With no remedy available currently and a possible vaccine far on the horizon, the virus has become more of an economic catastrophe than a health crisis. Protective lockdowns have brought the wheels of our economy to a grinding halt. Unfortunately, this decision has driven masses to death, if not by COVID-19 itself, then by consequent hunger. The saving grace is the low mortality and high recovery rates in Nepal.

The young Nepali manager is witnessing the scenario with horror. Experts assert that the worst is yet to come. India and many western countries are buckling under the onslaught of a second or third wave of COVID-19. Epidemiological studies hint at the emergence of deadlier viruses in the future, what with mankind exploiting nature relentlessly. Wildlife-based viruses are all set to invade our cities. Let us not forget that this virus entered the human system as bat and pangolin meat flooded Chinese wet markets. Sanitary measures are stricter now but one cannot alter the dietary habits of the world's most populous country easily. As they say, anything which moves is edible, not only in China but in many other South East Asian countries as well. It is a matter of culture stretching back to millennia.

With despair being the reigning sentiment, the young Nepali manager is evaluating rapidly deteriorating businesses with scepticism, doubt and distrust. As jobs vanish and salaries get slashed the executive is discovering his dreams getting dashed. The deep-rooted belief of a job for a lifetime is turning into a chimera. I am not surprised that youngsters have started blaming companies and their promoters. In a country where big business has never been given its pride of place, such a blame game is obvious. The ruling Leftist dispensation and its followers, even if unwittingly, strengthen this mentality. However, the corporate world has always been a soft target even in capitalist and free market economies.

Blame if you must but do suggest solutions as well, I say. Instead, I come across only deathly silence. This speechlessness speaks volumes about the state of affairs in Nepal. Breaching trust is easy; rebuilding it is difficult, very difficult.

Managers need to be rational while also keeping the faith. Only faith will offer hope of better times. Unbiased analysis will make youngsters understand the root cause of the present crisis. The two together will equip them to give their best when better times return and make their companies prosper again. Enterprises and managers are not mutually exclusive. They fall and rise together. Their destinies are intertwined. One and one can make eleven.

Women Deserve Legitimate Opportunities

February 2021

Kamala Harris was sworn in on 20 January 2021 as the first woman Vice President in American history as well as the first woman of African, American and Indian lineage. She reached the coveted position breaking barriers and glass ceilings which had denied women their rightful due ever since the formation of USA.

Harris's rise was rather heartwarming for civil society and saner elements in the US which witnessed a most violent and shameful transition of power from outgoing President Donald Trump who still remains blind to the stark public mandate against him. Other factors apart, her rise to power brought a glow to the sullen faces of most non-white Americans; this is not to say that she does not enjoy any 'white' support. However, many in South Asia are unable to comprehend the ecstatic welcome of Kamala Harris in the US. After all, India, Sri Lanka, Pakistan, Myanmar and Israel in West Asia have seen extended regimes headed by women. In fact, we found it surprising that the 'advanced and modern' US was a laggard in this respect till Kamala Harris rose despite her obstacles.

Politics apart, the US has been the hub of women's emancipation and empowerment. They have scaled the most difficult of heights in most domains including corporate business, entrepreneurship, education, science and technology, defence, literature, art and culture. If you have the will, then you have the highest possibility of carving a way for yourself in USA.

Unfortunately, we can't say the same for Nepal and neighbouring countries. Advances in politics are not reflected in other spheres of our life. Gender discrimination in Nepal remains heavily weighed against our girls and women. There has been a spurt in laws formulated to promise equality and equity to women, but deeply entrenched social mindsets easily overwhelm government and legislative endeavour.

Let us now focus on Nepali women's place in the business space. What is the shortest and most sustainable way of enhancing the participation of Nepalese women in business? Doubt over the need to do so is of utmost relevance. One wonders whether women are really cut out for cut-throat business. Let us go into the recent past. The country's most major companies and conglomerates had humble beginnings. The seeds were sown by determined entrepreneurs in place and time which were not the most hospitable. Those dedicated to business survived and thrived. Many more fell by the wayside. That is the way and nature of business. Successful business persons created wealth and employment for thousands. They built Nepal's economic spine at their own risk. Mind you, the private sector had to fend for itself unlike public sector undertakings as it did not have unaccounted access to public tax. So the challenges were daunting.

However, even after tasting success, many thriving companies have had to be on their toes. While the COVID-19 pandemic has shaken the roots of Nepali and global business, it's also becoming a question of sheer survival. All the more commendable that women who are trying to venture into business today deserve a salute from existing companies because they are beginning with a gender handicap in a strongly patriarchal society.

Let's scan some data. Women own merely 14 per cent of the firms registered in Nepal. Lack of finance and share in immovable property compels them to hunt for bare minimum seed capital. Bereft of collateral they are unable to raise funds. This being the scenario, women cannot showcase even technical expertise which is vital alongside networking for support from banks. This gender gap can be bridged. But very few are willing to invest in bringing women up to the desired level. This is despite the fact that heads of most banks and even CEOs of foreign companies operating in Nepal have a high opinion of our women managers' honesty, integrity, work quality and sense of responsibility. The lady head of a Nepali bank had no qualms in telling at a conference that default by women was close to zero and they were willing to pay more to the lender. Companies led and owned by women were making 10 to 15 per cent higher profit than businesses owned by men, she added.

An entrepreneurial spirit forms the root of corporate business. But we also know that entrepreneurship is subject to high mortality. Gestation period and break even can be painfully long. Scalability is difficult and most enterprises get stuck after reaching a certain level. It is here that major Nepali corporates can play a game changing role. They should head to the campuses and recruit the best managerial talent from among female students. As our economy recovers from the pandemic's blow and employment grows, corporates should start inducting more and more female professionals. Their capability and commitment as corporate managers is unquestionable. Companies are hurting themselves and society by neglecting women.

Women do not need doles, they deserve legitimate opportunities. Let us not overvalue men and undervalue women. We have done that for ages. It's time to be fair. Is that too difficult?

Humane Managers For Troubled Times

March 2021

I feel more than bemused when people talk of the post-pandemic economic scenario. Is COVID-19 really dead? Has it ultimately bid goodbye to the planet? Will the recently launched vaccines triumph over the most deadly virus in living memory? Are we certain about the vaccines' efficacy and longevity? And what about the side effects of these virus fighters created in a mighty hurry? Listen to the experts carefully and you will find that none of them has a definite and confident answer to these normal queries haunting the common man.

We are aware that the COVID-19 virus is fast mutating and is staging a comeback in several countries where it had started fading. There is also talk of mini and micro pandemics hitting current and new geographies any time. COVID-19, thy name is uncertainty and you are far from gone. Perhaps, you have decided to stay for good and torment us in different forms.

This being the reality, it is ridiculous to talk of a post-pandemic economic scenario even if the *HBR*, McKinsey and other reputed academic and practising business platforms think so. Optimism and hope are essential but not at the cost of hard reality.

Yet we need to live on with as little fear as possible. The latest and more horrific crisis overshadows the lesser ones we confronted in the past. The world has faced and overcome recessions and economic downturns that hit us with alarming regularity. Major recessions have been rocking global commerce almost every decade. The sub-prime crisis of 2007–09 and the dot-com bust at the beginning of the century are still fresh in our minds. So it does make sense to pick up the pieces from the past and learn to live with long-term recession. We must remember that while recessions may stop making it to media headlines after some time, their deleterious impact lasts a long time with some of the damage remaining undone forever. Yet we need to move on. So what is the learning from the past?

A regular check-up of your company's health is no less significant than your own medical check-up. Honestly scrutinize inefficiencies in your product or service offerings. The COVID-19 induced upheaval has shown that economic ups and downs are now more imminent than ever. Let's not forget that COVID-19 is still raging and causing mayhem. It is also time to assess your HR strength to maintain or exceed current output. However, resorting to layoffs as the sole HR intervention is not wise; it causes apprehension among your current and potential employees.

The honest scrutiny based on hard data will enable you to identify the pain points in your company. What should be done to make the organization better equipped to sail through troubled times which are set to become the new normal in business? Are some employees engaged in doing repetitive tasks? Is the company focusing too much on low-margin products and services? Changes are called for. Go in for job sharing. Employees engaged in low-margin activities can be moved to the company's profit centres. Such changes may lead to unwarranted publicity. Honest and transparent HR interventions with the affected workforce can pre-empt this possibility. The nobility of your intentions and actions will keep your reputation intact and protect your business.

It may sound counter-intuitive but the fact is that employee-linked changes can 'maximize' your existing teams even during recession and slowdown. How?

Writing in HR-centric website Insperity.com, Jenisse Chaffold provides some tips. While existing leaders should obviously be encouraged and reassured, the company should try to identify its undiscovered leaders and empower them. Provide them bigger responsibilities. Employees should be told that their hard work and loyalty during these troubled times will not go unappreciated. This will ensure high morale and consistent output.

Such an approach needs to be accompanied by intangible benefits to employees, particularly those entrusted with higher responsibility. It needs to be understood that an individual employee is under greater stress than the company during recessionary times. He suffers financial, emotional and personal family-linked issues. So, mere monetary compensation will not motivate him. Flexible timing, work-from-home opportunities are known to ease employee pain.

Managers should be trained to deal with mental and emotional health issues being faced by the employees. Mental health challenges can affect the entire workplace.

Qualified HR professionals can play a big role in this context. To make the company recession-proof one needs to think long term. Your HR team should be well trained in communication and risk mitigation. This needs to be done proactively and not when the sky is falling on your head. People run companies. An empathetic and healing HR hand can equip managers, staff and workers to tackle terrible troubles tactfully.

Lessons From COVID-19 For the Top Brass

June 2021

COVID-19 has been plaguing the planet for over a year and a half. The end of the killer pandemic is nowhere in sight. Most facets of our life have been turned topsy-turvy. So it would be criminally clichéd to ask whether the business leadership style too has changed during these catastrophic times. It may though be pertinent to ask as to who has adapted better to the changed business scenario: the top brass or budding managers?

By its very nature, youth is more amenable to change. Unburdened by the legacy of the past and enthused by the promise of a bright future, young managers have always been in the forefront of embracing modern ways. But the green signal has to come from the top. Unfortunately, the big bosses are too steeped in their antediluvian management and business style to shake off the past and catch up with the times.

But COVID-19 is now shaking the big bosses out of their slumber. It is becoming increasingly obvious that companies which had adopted digitalization early have not only coped with the current crisis better but are also way ahead of the competition. Proactive change in leadership styles is the secret of their success. Google is a stellar example of what I would call a revolution. We are now witnessing a part of the Google act happening around us in the form of remote or work-from-home working.

Did we have to wait for a worldwide pandemic to adopt a work style which enamours us today? Too large a section of the top business leadership would still judge young managers by office attendance, rather than productivity. By stubbornly sticking to their outmoded thinking in this disease-ravaged time, the bosses are also putting the lives of managers at grave risk. These 'pucca' top managers are always found swearing by 'dhandha' and mocking modern management which is more empirical, measurable, data and welfare-driven.

Doesn't remote working make more sense even from the 'profit-only' perspective of these 'pucca' bosses? You save big money on office real estate. Conveyance expenses get drastically reduced. Young managers have more time and energy to focus on their real job. The list goes on and on though with the caveat that remote working cannot be all pervasive particularly for blue-collar workers in manufacturing workshops. To optimize benefits from remote working, the top managers—who are invariably senior in years—need to change their outlook. Gone are the days when micro-management used to be the in-thing and work used to be extracted through fear and threat of punishment. A well-qualified young manager certainly does not relish his immediate boss staring down his shoulders all the time. Why this lack of trust? Is it just because the bosses were treated this way by their higher-ups in the typical saas bahu (mother-in-law vs. daughter-in-law) manner?

Even basic knowledge of modern HRD techniques would help. There are tested and proven ways of enhancing engagement of managers, especially young ones, with the company. Measurement of performance can be made more objective and task-relevant through techniques like a balanced scorecard. I am not advocating escape from accountability for young executives. However, their invasive monitoring should be a big 'no'.

But are the old economy chiefs willing to give up hierarchy and run a flatter organization? If they have not so far, then they will have to now, not only because modern systems are bearing better results but also because the days of whip-wielding slave masters are gone. New ways of optimizing human resources are emerging and are being lapped up by enlightened top bosses and companies. It is plain as day that only the top bosses can lead the way to change, particularly in our part of the world. We are still living in semi-feudal times. However eager and enthusiastic young managers may be regarding modern management, they can do little till those who hold the purse strings choose to listen. So the prime task of upcoming managers, management gurus and B-schools is to promote and propagate the advantages of remote functioning and a host of allied changes for business.

Or shall we wait for more cataclysmic occurrences before we are compelled to adopt the enlightened path?

B-school Lessons From the 'Street'

July 2021

The informal business sector rules our streets, pavements, village bazaars and the remotest of locations. Operating out of tiny shops, tarpaulin-covered structures, bamboo kiosks, wheel carts and even bicycles, these small businesses cater to the bulk of our day-to-day needs.

Yet the informal sector remains unhonoured and unsung. Youngsters, particularly those who are privileged to receive some education, prefer to remain unemployed and thus dependent on their ageing parents rather than join the informal sector. Why? Our society looks down upon 'petty' work. Our education system has taught us anything but dignity of labour. No wonder small-level entrepreneurship is looked down upon.

Being largely unregistered and unregulated, informal businesses do not easily lend themselves to accurate data collection by government authorities. They, therefore, miss out on availing of whatever meagre government facilities do exist for them. According to an International Labour Organization estimate, over 70 per cent of Nepal's economically active population is engaged in the informal sector business. And this number is rising!

A World Bank report (October 2020) proclaimed that informal workers will be the worst hit by the seemingly unstoppable COVID-19 pandemic as they have no social security and face extreme poverty and exploitation. Economists are of the view that urban and semi-urban informal enterprises are placed worse than rural units which can draw sustenance from their farms. That is why the World Bank has been advocating universal social protection. Governments and local authorities cannot leave the vulnerable sections of society to fend for themselves especially during the COVID-19 crisis, which has deeply scarred our and the South Asian economy.

A February 2021 report by the Nepal Economic Forum asserts that 84.6 per cent of Nepal's labour force ekes out a living from informal enterprises. The figure includes not just workers but also unregistered business owners like street vendors. This oppressed lot is unable to avail of any social security benefits or formal financing. Relief available to formal employees remains a mirage for informal workers, the report asserts. Yet the informal sector constitutes the biggest business environment in the world. Surveys show informal units are growing globally. Their domain is large but their contribution to the GDP is relatively low. For example, in India 90 per cent of the labour force is involved in the informal sector but its share in the country's GDP is just 50 per cent. This is a sad reality.

Predictions that this marginalized sector will only grow add to our concerns and worry. Will more and more of our educated youth (read management graduates) be compelled to become informal sector entrepreneurs? The predicament is not unlikely considering our economic model wherein growth will happen only by slashing jobs. Technology—artificial intelligence, machine learning et al—is fast becoming the biggest enemy of working humans. It is in this context that we need to study the survival skills of the informal sector which has been battling assaults by heartless technology for a long time. The secret lies in the informal businesses' agility, ingenuity, innovativeness and the ability to take double-quick decisions. These attributes come naturally to them because their necks are always on the chopping block. They change so that they do not perish.

The return on investment in the informal sector is way higher than the formal sector. Also, the informal sector ensures equitable distribution of profit down the supply chain. The profit margin of the ultimate seller is quite slim as she shares the proceeds with a number of persons involved in creating the product, namely, momos, noodles, dal-bhat, samosas, etc. There is amazing fluidity in the informal sector's market mix. The same person is seen selling different things during different festival seasons without having ever heard of Enterprise Resource Planning (ERP) or System, Applications & Products (SAP). Compare that to the long time—five to seven years—taken by the formal sector to change a product line. There are many street vendors who sell 'chana' (roasted gram) to joggers around parks in the morning and move to liquor shops in the evening to cater to a separate customer base. While the street flower or toy seller can decide to offer even a 50 per cent discount to his customer any time, a corporate manager has to go way up the management chain to get even a 5 per cent price cut approved.

While companies prattle unceasingly about gender diversity, the phenomenon has been a reality in street, pavement and hole-in-the-wall businesses forever. The street is a free trainer for aspiring managers. Go, walk it!

Greed Continues To Breed

August 2021

COVID-19 has scared the wits out of us. Even the smartest don't know what has hit the planet. No wonder the fear of God has struck even atheists and agnostics.

After two years of the ongoing pandemic, we should supposedly be a fairly sobered lot today. But are we? At least, the super-rich and corporate behemoths are not. News about big financial frauds keep trickling in from all corners of the world. White-collar crime, the most debilitating and rampant offence perpetrated by the rich against the masses, continues to flourish. Greed continues to breed!

Why is it so? Why do the rich continue to indulge in financial misappropriations and rackets even when their next seven generations are taken care of? They possess more than what they can use and enjoy. *Par dil hai ki manta nahin* (yet the heart remains unfulfilled). Has greed become genetic to humankind?

What is greed's genesis? Perhaps in the unicellular amoeba which god knows when started devouring its counterparts to grow, split and develop into complex living beings, including the human species. Have we inherited the amoeba's greed to grow? Is that propensity still embedded in us, driving our behaviour to acquire and possess whatever we can even after millions or maybe billions of years? But this sounds rather fanciful now. So let us move to matters which seem practical and pragmatic in current times.

From childhood, we are inspired and coaxed by elders to become 'bada aadmi' – the big guy who owns wealth, wields authority and is therefore usually held in high esteem by society, or even feared. But how many parents tell their children to rise in life only through honest means? No wonder, the child grows up determined to become a bada aadmi by whatever means possible. That is where greed, corruption, dishonesty, forgery, bribery, etc. come into play. The growing adolescent does not even realize that he is straying from the ethical path. After all, he sees 'successful' elders becoming 'great' and 'honourable' walking the dubious path. The irony is that alongside we also bemoan the decadence prevailing in society. Isn't it all of our own making? We create a perfect environment for our progeny to imbibe all that is vile and immoral. Why do we then seek the culprits elsewhere when we are ourselves to blame? This is yet another trait of human chicanery so much in evidence today.

On top of that, white-collar criminals, including corporate barons, have the gall to say that moneymaking is just smart play with no adverse repercussions for general society. Can crimes like fraud, bribery, Ponzi schemes, embezzlement, insider trading, cybercrime, intellectual property infringement, racketeering, money laundering, identity theft, forgery, etc. leave the common man unaffected? This is a myth assiduously perpetuated by white-collar criminals to ward off public ire and be seen as lily-white. Fortunately, this does not happen and people see through the charade.

Let us dwell upon some corporate malpractices which often put otherwise clean and well-meaning young executives in a quandary. In the absence of clear-cut corporate governance policies, junior managers at times fail to distinguish between right and wrong. They become all the more perplexed when they find hanky-panky happening around them getting ignored by the top management. Such ambiguous behaviour is perceived as endorsement by executives who are still wet behind the ears. Corruption creeps in unwittingly. The gate to ethical transgressions gets opened. A well-known German engineering MNC had tweaked its accounting methods to organize bribe payments in millions of dollars. It was seen as the company's business model by employees.

A more than hundred-year-old retail banking and financial services company in the USA devised an incentive plan which allowed thousands of its employees to cheat customers till as late as four years ago.

Often aggressive goals set by companies compel managers to adopt unethical means. The 'do-what-it-takes' approach pushes managers into immoral terrain. Arrogance following long runs of malpractices makes many corporates and their employees believe that they are above the law. Most of them are caught one day but by then they have inflicted massive damage on themselves and society at large.

Industrial psychologists have repeatedly highlighted lack of empathy among the rich for commoners and social welfare policies. Yet leading rating agencies have been backing companies which have repeatedly or rather habitually fallen prey to greed. The greed breed is growing. It's time for the correct corporates to create an anti-greed creed.

The Triumph of Humanity

September 2021

Oh, how a tiny news report tucked away in a foreign newspaper can set you thinking afresh! Yes, this is what happened to me when I chanced upon the news quoting Dutch historian Rutger Bregman at a literary festival. The headline read: 'You have to believe that humans are (mostly) good.'

Well, this may not sound very surprising to us in our part of the world. But believe me, the West thinks rather differently. Western thought and culture are based on the premise that humans are basically selfish. Ever since Eve committed the 'original sin' in the Garden of Eden by eating the forbidden fruit from the tree, mankind has been treated as an intrinsic sinner.

No wonder western corporate philosophy too is driven by the belief 'that deep down people are just nasty and selfish or even monsters'. The quoted portion comes from Bregman whose book *Humankind: A Hopeful History* (2019) cocks a snook at the established order in governments, businesses, elites and all those who actually run the world even as the common citizen thinks that he empowers and controls the top guns through his democratic right to vote. Bregman finds the citizen's perception entirely misconceived. And therefore, the young Dutch historian has been taking up the cudgels against the real ruling class at any given opportunity, including platforms like the Davos summit.

Bregman's bestselling books, including *Utopia for Realists: How We Can Build the Ideal World* (2014), have raised many hackles in the top corporate crust, which is a vigorous votary and practitioner of the command-and-control model. The bosses have no hope of any good coming on its own from their teams. Pessimism is deeply entrenched in their psyche thanks to the ancient 'original sin' tale. Such doubt and suspicion can only serve as a death wish which smothers spontaneous optimism and motivation in the working class.

But this deeply flawed management model remains in currency and that too beyond the western business hemisphere as well. Why is it so? After all, our philosophical and theological roots are so different.

The simple reason is that underdeveloped and developing countries like ours have imbibed the western models lock, stock and barrel. The razzle and dazzle of the wealthy West have blinded us. Instead of picking and choosing what suits our culture and system, we have imbibed the western way of business management in totality. So, are we saying that our heritage of trust and confidence in our own people and workers is bunkum?

I firmly believe that management strategies based on fundamental mistrust in colleagues and co-workers can only spell disaster. Why would a team trust its manager who has no faith in them? The Orient is a different world. Interpersonal relationships can make or mar businesses. Unlike the West, a business enterprise is viewed as an extension of the family here. Transactional relationships cannot, rather, do not last long. Look around and you will see how countries like Japan, South Korea, Singapore and Taiwan rose virtually from the rubble by sticking to their own social and management ethos. Vietnam, Bangladesh and the Philippines too are riding astride the upward curve by doing things their own way. The human touch offered by one's own tradition and culture cannot be supplanted by entirely foreign and alien ways.

To quote young Bregman again: 'So what is this radical idea? That most people, deep down, are pretty decent... It's when crisis hits—when the bombs fall or the floodwaters rise—that we humans become our best selves.' Had humankind been visceral sinners we would not have witnessed the exemplary cooperation and collaboration among countries against the raging COVID-19 pandemic. It is because of the fundamental goodness in humans that extreme poverty, child mortality, child labour, famines, wars, deaths in natural disasters have plummeted over the last several decades, Bregman asserts, while at the same time calling upon the elites to do more (read higher taxes) for society which has let their coffers bloat. The elites find such suggestions incendiary because, as Bregman claims, they have turned shameless. With economic inequality growing by the day, the real sinners need to be named and shamed. Why blame the entire human race? That would definitely be inhuman. No, sinful!

Climate Crisis Is Real and NOW!

November 2021

Clear and present crises often overshadow bigger dangers lurking in the background. The global panic caused by the COVID-19 pandemic has diverted our attention from many other lethal predators.

The Wuhan virus killer has claimed over 4.7 million lives across the planet till 30 September 2021. It has wrecked societies and economies. Governments are being hailed or hauled over the coals depending on their good or bad performance in the ongoing battle against the lethal virus which kept reincarnating in deadlier forms over the last two years.

Compare this to the under-reported and largely neglected figures about the air pollution toll provided recently by the World Health Organization (WHO). The global organization says that almost the entire world breathes air that breaches WHO guideline limits. Result: almost seven million deaths worldwide every year with low- and middle-income countries being the worst sufferers. It is obvious that air pollution and the resultant climate change are far bigger killers than COVID-19. The two have been stalking the earth for years, creating deadlier records with time. Yet, compared to the frenetic fight against

COVID-19 our concern about climate change seems rather muted.

Why should this be so?

Is it because a club of 100 investor-and-state-owned fossil fuel (coal, petroleum and natural gas) companies account for 70 per cent of the world's historical greenhouse gas (GHG) emissions? These mighty corporations have the wherewithal to create their own narrative to run the way they do. It was estimated in 2019 that the world's five largest publicly owned oil and gas companies spent about $200 million annually to influence climate policy to their advantage. The world suffers as it hurtles towards disaster. The corporations forget that they are part of the planet and environmental disasters won't play lovey-dovey with them.

Writing in the *HBR* in January 2020, Elliott Hyman asserted that business behemoths tend to place the responsibility for fighting climate change on individual consumers, 'conveniently ignoring the disproportionate climate impact of corporate interests... At the current rate of global greenhouse gas emissions, climate change could displace two billion people due to rising ocean levels...all before (year) 2100.'

Hyman took up the cudgels against the corporations with the following data-backed argument: '... individual actions have minute effects relative to these (GHG) emissions—average American households produce only 8.1 metric tons of carbon dioxide out of a total of over 33 billion tons globally. Fossil fuel interests spend billions on climate science denial to mislead the public about the truth behind the crisis and push the misperception that through individual actions alone climate change can be stopped.' The assiduous manipulation of the climate narrative drives even the common man to harbour serious doubts about the truthfulness of climate change. Add to this the tribe of pompous politicians like former US President Donald Trump who mock climate change as a myth and "fake science". Trump may have lost to Joe Biden but he had hordes of diehard supporters who caused mayhem in the White House on his defeat. It, indeed, takes all kinds to make the world.

There is no dearth of dirty tricks in the corporate bag. It is being argued that tackling climate change is not economically feasible. Economists differ. They say that even 1 per cent of the global GDP can make a considerable difference. Neglect now and later will only push up the cost, with current and ensuing suffering being a certainty. Mark Maslin, professor of Earth System Science, University College London, writes, 'But if we don't act now, by 2050 it would cost over 20 per cent of world GDP... What the climate change deniers also forget to tell you is that they are protecting a fossil fuel industry that receives \$5.2 trillion in annual subsidies... This amounts to six per cent of global GDP.'

Professor Maslin quoted International Monetary Fund (IMF) estimates, which claim that efficient fossil fuel pricing would lower global carbon emissions by 28 per cent, fossil fuel air pollution deaths by 46 per cent, and increase government revenue by 3.8 per cent of the country's GDP.

Why can't corporates be sensible and humane for a change?

Compassion Makes Good Business

December 2021

Cane versus compassion. Whip versus wisdom. What drives business better? What ensures longevity, profitability and sustainability of a company? What promotes employee loyalty?

These are some of the questions that continue to trouble business biggies. Ever since the inception of modern business there has been no dearth of business owners and top managers betting in favour of coercive measures for growing business. Factories and shop floors have, for centuries, witnessed the worst treatment of human labour. Such inhuman treatment has found ample reflection in global literature that still brings tears to our eyes. But the feudal era, when industries were striking roots, is gradually on its way out though the mindset still lingers in pockets. In-depth research in industrial psychology and human resource management is bringing to light hitherto neglected systems. Business is becoming more humane. Simultaneously, it is being recognized that compassion and business success are compatible.

The trauma of the COVID-19 pandemic is far from over even two years after it broke out. But this period saw a greater focus on compassion. Nobel Peace Prize winner and foremost leader of

Tibetan Buddhism, the Dalai Lama describes compassion as 'sense of commitment, responsibility and respect towards the other.' Words like compassion, grace, kindness are generally associated with the spiritual world, which is deemed to be way apart from the worldly realm. It is heartening to find that the two spheres are getting closer and that purely profit-driven business is regaining sublime moorings.

The question is whether compassion and business realities can travel together and for how long. Now that COVID-19 is on the decline in some parts of the world, managers are wondering whether flexibilities (delayed deadlines, relaxed goals, lowered productivity, etc.) extended to employees during the pandemic's peak should be continued or recalibrated. Will employees take advantage of the benefits offered in COVID-19 times?

Jane Dutton, professor at the University of Michigan's Ross School of Business and co-author of *Awakening Compassion at Work*, states, 'Being compassionate doesn't mean you have to lower your standards.' The professor instead stresses upon combining compassion and accountability.

In most such discussions, we lose sight of the hit which the mental health of the staff has taken because of the unprecedented COVID-19 pandemic. They have lost faith not only in themselves but even in the best of business managements, governments, medical facilities and local administrations. After all, the pandemic had brought everybody down to their knees. Even as the deadly disease continues to rage in some parts of the world, vaccine politics has dealt a lethal blow to the underprivileged and the marginalized. Yet, vaccine pharma giants are raking in obscene profits. The tragic scenario is making the common man all the more vulnerable. Emotional health has taken a hard knock as uncertainty looms large in front of most of us. It's time for businesses to practise compassion as best as they can.

So what should businesses do?

First, change your thought processes. You extended flexibility to your employees and executives, not leniency, during the pandemic. Don't look down upon your team; do not be condescending.

Top management should not be driven by stereotypes and prejudices. There is no direct correlation between the management's tough measures and superior performance by the staff. Research shows that threatening behaviour stifles innovation as employees continue to focus only on what they already know.

Jacob Hirsh, associate professor at the University of Toronto, has been quoted thus: 'At a purely instrumental strategic level, you're not going to get the results you want if you add stress to people's lives.' A manager should ensure a psychologically safe workplace for his team. Compassion propels employees to give back more to the organization. Fear does not work as the key most of the time.

All this is not to say that underperformance is not an issue. But it needs to be treated differently in these tumultuous times. Understand and identify the issues being faced by the underperformer. Meet them individually or in groups, but with an open mind. You will be able to know what is hurting them and how they can be motivated to get back on track. But that will happen only if you are driven by compassion.

Green Shoots in Nepal's Entrepreneurship

January 2022

The boy was at his wits' end. Having just stepped into his teens, he was flustered by a common advice being piled upon him from all quarters, from neighbours to stationery seller to vegetable vendor to milkman, and, of course, from most relatives. *'Achchhi naukri karna'* (Get a good job). The trauma continued till the education minister visited his class. The nervous teacher, apparently to impress the minister, squeaked, *'Achchhi naukri karna.'* But even before the boy could utter a word, the minister stated, *'Achchhi naukri dena'.* (Provide good jobs). 'If all of you want to take up jobs only, then who will create and provide new jobs?' The class broke into a cheer.

Obviously, a myth had been shattered.

This is the gist of an advertisement running in most Indian TV channels currently. Sponsored by the government of the national capital territory of Delhi, the campaign hits out at the mad race for secure government jobs in our part of the world. Those who reject the trodden path to launch their own enterprises from scratch are the ones who create job opportunities and wealth for society. Yet the same society, caught in its traditional and backward thinking, denies due respect to these entrepreneurs. Recognition comes to these bravehearts after years of toil and struggle.

The TV advertisement I talked of is a testimony of the changing times. The government is fast realizing that the days of government jobs for all are gone; they will not return. Growing countries are now actively following the principle of less government and more governance. Advanced and wealthy nations had understood and imbibed this fundamental postulate way before. That is why they are where they are. They endured the pain of entrepreneurship, failed and fumbled, time and again, but got back on their feet. And then came the gain that got spread across society, not by way of mere jobs in their growing enterprises but by bolstering the entrepreneurial spirit. If he (the entrepreneur) can do it, then why can't we. Societies and countries started thinking thus and gained prosperity, the entrepreneurial way.

I find this vital energy cutting across age barriers now. Earlier when we discussed someone's career or future the person being talked about, generally, used to be in his or her twenties. But now even persons in their forties or fifties are seeking to plough a new furrow for themselves.

Lately, I managed to scrape out time for some quality TV watching. Sony TV has recently launched a programme called *Shark Tank India*, a franchise of its western version. The programme provides a platform to start-ups and aspiring entrepreneurs for live interaction with venture capitalists who have a successful launch record. So far, I have seen entrepreneurs from 16 to 50+ years of age discussing and sharing their business proposals and experience with venture capitalists. They seek funding against equity in their proposed businesses. It is not just money that the entrepreneurs are looking for. Many a time, they settle for a lesser investment offer if they feel that the funder's experience, contacts, passion, etc. may add greater value to their enterprise. On the spot, decisions are taken and cheques are issued to the entrepreneurs, much to their delight. Many aspirants return empty-handed, but considerably enriched by the advice from the highly experienced venture capitalists, some of whom have built $2 billion brands.

Enterprises may appear to be the stuff of dreams to some, but they are hardly so for those who combine passion with pragmatism. Today, we indeed hear of more than one unicorn (a privately held start-up company with a value of over $1 billion) making its presence known in the business world every month. That may seem a lot but we need not forget that thousands of start-ups fall by the wayside.

The COVID-19 pandemic has been imparting new lessons to us every day. Entrepreneurs need to be all the more vigilant about them. Are your start-ups and also your team nimble, flexible and responsive to the new and emerging needs of the market? Are you ready and equipped to make changes in your pricing, marketing, staffing, warehousing, etc.? Remember that all this will be possible only if you are able to lead a culture change in your enterprise. No less important is admission of the fact that all business factors are not under your control at all times, and more so during a global health catastrophe. So, brainstorm and discover the factors that are within your control. Focus on them. That is the practical way of saving and growing your enterprise and also keeping intact your faith in entrepreneurship.

Righteous vs Smart

February 2022

I don't exactly remember when I started addressing Madhav Kant Sahay as 'Madho Babu'. It perhaps happened gradually and unknowingly as I witnessed him gaining knowledge and wisdom, and most importantly, displaying honesty and integrity. However, these virtues were also accompanied by an exaggerated sense of self-righteousness in him.

Madho Babu would not budge from what *he* thought was correct. Though he did follow the right path most of the time, he was rather unwilling to amend his ways even at the cost of annoying his superiors. We know there is scarce space for such persons today. So, Madho Babu did rise in his managerial career but not to the extent he could have.

This is a sad episode from Madho Babu's short stint as the career communication general manager in an MNC with its Indian headquarters in Mumbai. The tenure could have been happier and longer had Madho Babu gone by the dictates of his immediate boss who happened to be the company's managing director (MD).

Usually, the corporate communication head reports directly to the organization's chairman or MD because he/she has to be aware of all the developments and plans of the company and needs to interact with a host of stakeholders—from employees to government and regulatory bodies, banks, dealers, suppliers/vendors, current and potential customers, and, of course, the ubiquitous media.

Let's get back to Madho Babu's entry in the new company in Mumbai. He approached the MD and sought to know his expectations from the corporate communication department. Strangely, the boss had nothing to share. Madho Babu returned from the MD's office carrying a load of past annual reports, an almost ancient book on the company's history and several marketing brochures. The MD did voice his desire for the maintenance of the company's reputation but also made it clear that he would be able to spare some time for just one media interview a month.

Back at his desk, Madho Babu faced another shock. His team disclosed that the company's in-house quarterly journal, which used to be distributed in the company's fourteen manufacturing plants across India, had not been published for nine months. It transpired that Madho Babu's predecessor, a marketing professional with little writing and journalistic experience, was engaged in producing a book on sustainable manufacturing all this while at the expense of core communication activities. How could a multinational behemoth, which had acquired the Indian company only a few years ago, ignore its most important stakeholders—thousands of blue-collar workers spread across its huge factories in India? Wouldn't this affect work culture integration?

Madho Babu also found that most communication work had come to a standstill because the team members had no corporate communication skills and had got their jobs before the MNC took over through recommendations and trade union pressure.

Madho Babu again sought the MD's ears. The MD was aware of the situation but did not relish tackling problems. However, he would not authorize Madho Babu either to set his team in order. Also, the MD would often order communication staffers to carry out his personal errands like arranging tickets for his personal foreign trips or buy gifts for his family.

Left to himself, Madho Babu burnt the midnight oil and published the long languishing in-house journals in a far more interesting and employee-centric manner. He wrote articles on behalf of the MD and got them published in leading national newspapers. This naturally invited acclaim from the company's top managers. Top business papers started writing about the company. Even the MD had to acknowledge Madho Babu's contribution in the intra-company net.

Madho Babu, foolishly enough, retorted that much more could be done if the MD acted professionally. The big boss was not used to such candour. The very same evening, he told Madho Babu that he was not up to the challenges the company faced. Madho Babu asked him to be specific. The MD found the entreaty below his dignity. Madho Babu was out within three months of joining the company, though his name remained on the rolls for another three months and he continued to receive salary.

But no sooner had the six months expired that Madho Babu's predecessor was back in the company, happy with the team he had built honouring recommendations from influential quarters. The corporate communications team became the personal fiefdom of the MD doing his biddings, right or wrong.

It is another issue that the company's board sniffed mischief and showed the door to the MD within a year. But why do the likes of Madho Babu suffer? Are they not *smart* enough?

The Creation of Intrapreneurs

March 2022

COVID-19 is on the wane, but it has left behind a humongous trail of deaths and disruptions in life as well as business across the globe. And, of course, the fear of its return in another form continues to haunt us.

Yet, resilient as the human species is, it is trying to bounce back. Focusing on business, battered and bruised companies are trying to get back on their feet. But the million-dollar question that continues to loom is—can we pre-empt the debacle such as the one that was just unleashed by the unprecedented pandemic by continuing with our established ways of business? Though this is a top-of-the-mind issue bothering the business world globally, I would rather focus on the prevailing situation in Nepal.

The country needs to evolve and execute a new model that will pre-empt recurrence of crises, like the one triggered by COVID-19. Nepal is not exactly known for its HRD practices. In fact, we hardly have any system in place when it comes to HRD, which is practiced most arbitrarily. We forget that in a resource-scarce country like ours, only the rank and file of an enterprise can bring about effective and discernible change. We do not have recourses to technology that can bring about societal change at the ground level. Lack of funds is not the only stumbling block in the acquisition of technology; we do not have people to make use of it efficiently.

Talk to industrialists and businessmen in Nepal and you will come across a common complaint: salaried employees lack the vigour and passion of entrepreneurs. The grouse has more than a grain of truth in it. Those who are running our big enterprises today were entrepreneurs till not so long ago. They and their ancestors have experienced the blood and toil that goes into the creation of a company or conglomerate. However, their current success camouflages their failures and fumbling, over the past few decades, from the new generation. No wonder the captains of industry in Nepal find their white and blue-collar teams nowhere as committed as themselves.

Having said this, I must simultaneously admit that entrepreneurs have the same grievance in the advanced world too. But they have come up with a solution that has been doing fairly well for their companies. I am talking of Intrapreneurship.

The American Heritage Dictionary defines an intrapreneur as 'a person within a large corporation who takes direct responsibility for turning an idea into a profitable finished product through assertive risk-taking and innovation.'

Lest there be any misunderstanding that an intrapreneur is usually a person innovating or inventing things only in information technology, artificial intelligence, machine learning and other high-tech areas, I should make it clear that I have all realms of business in mind. Why can ground-breaking innovation not happen in HRD, finance, accounting, manufacturing, logistics, industrial psychology, service processes, retail management and so on? The wheel runs smoothly only when each and every cog functions perfectly.

Thanks to the world-wide media, the new generation is aware of the changes in the global work arena. Many of them are imbued with the spirit of entrepreneurship, which they want to put into action within a company as employees. They are willing to take risks for rewards. They have the confidence to innovate and compete within their company to execute their ideas. Life-changing innovations that global business behemoths and recently emerging unicorns are flooding the world with are not the contribution of merely their renowned entrepreneurs and promoters. The successes we are witnessing today are the direct contribution of a large number of intrapreneurs working in these enlightened companies.

Are companies in Nepal willing to induct and encourage intrapreneurial talent? Are we willing to disrupt established hierarchies in companies and let these bright boys and girls change the face of our business? Yes, they may commit mistakes. However, show me one successful business tycoon who has not faltered in his business journey or does not err even now when he is on the top. The citadel of success is built upon the ruins of busts and debacles.

Identifying and embracing intrapreneurs is not an easy job though. In fact, we are not even willing to believe that there are youngsters who wish to join a company to identify real problems and solve them rather than to seek a safe and secure corporate cushion. They understand that solving problems and improving people's lives make great business. They are shakers and movers. They abhor the status quo. That is why they stand apart. We need to learn how to attract and retain youngsters with fire in their belly.

Forefront Education

May 2022

Though bordered by two giant neighbours, Nepal is geographically not a tiny nation. It spreads across an area of 147,516 square kilometres that has mountains, hills and plains. Yet, Nepal's population is below 30 million (three crore).

But it is highly disturbing that the country has failed to create employment and other work opportunities for the majority of its able-bodied male population. Though it is difficult to provide the exact number of Nepalis working abroad to keep families in proper shape back home, estimates suggest that 3.5 million to 8 million countrymen are eking out a living in India and around 6 million are working in countries like Qatar, Saudi Arabia, UAE, Malaysia, South Korea and Japan. Remittances sent by these Nepali workers account for 30 per cent of the country's GDP. This flow of funds from sons of the soil has kept the country, so to say, afloat and mitigated the poverty rate. The underprivileged and deprived class in the country is now able to create sustainable assets like permanent housing, giving a boost to the real estate industry. Children are being sent to better schools. Medical care is becoming affordable.

One wishes that this could continue but one foresees serious reservations on this score. The migration rush is yet another proof of the fact that Nepal, despite being an independent country all through its history, is still not able to offer sustainable living to its populace. With most able-bodied males compelled to toil in tough and pitiable circumstances in alien climates and climes, the agricultural sector has been dealt a massive blow. A net exporter of farm produce till the 1990s, Nepal has to today import food to feed its people. Overdependence on our migrant population brings in its trail unexpected vagaries. The COVID-19 pandemic witnessed our people rushing back to the homeland in the toughest of conditions. It was a humanitarian crisis for our workers abroad and an economic disaster at home. According to an estimate by the International Labour Organization, 1.6 million to 2 million jobs were disrupted in Nepal's wholesale and retail trade, manufacturing, construction, transport, food services and real estate sectors, to name just a few industries that were hurt the most.

The other concern about our hardworking migrant workers is also very grave. It is no secret that most of our boys seeking work abroad are not equipped with any competitive skills. So they have to engage in utter manual labour or semi-skilled work like welding, basic carpentry, etc. What is their competitive advantage? The ability and willingness to work in most inhospitable and tiring conditions with no regulatory benefits like provident fund, medical care and livable accommodation. And all this at lowly wages! It is a shame that our youth have to suffer this way to keep the home fires burning.

But will even this hellish avenue even be available to Nepal's young men as technology makes giant strides, and automation, artificial intelligence and machine learning hold the reins of human progress? Machines are advancing and pushing us out of many domains that were hitherto the exclusive reserves of human beings.

Though the debate over machines and jobs has been raging forever, the fact is that humans can survive only if they upgrade themselves to keep pace with technology, particularly information technology and its rapidly emerging off-shoots. There is no harm in seeking work abroad. That has been the way of international trade and travel for millennia. But why should we be driven to pick up the lowliest of jobs? Are we destined to be the coolies of the planet?

According to recent data from the United Nations Department of Economic and Social Affairs (DESA), by the year 2050 the earth's population will reach around 9.8 billion, with 6 billion people being of working age. Well over 70 million young people are already struggling to find decent jobs. It seems that the data does not include many who hold jobs but are actually under-employed. Either they do not have skills that the job market requires or their wages do not match their skills and qualifications.

One can say with a fair degree of conviction that the education system in under-developed countries, including Nepal, is hardly aligned with the needs of the world. Most degrees, diplomas and certificates are not worth the paper they are printed on. With this being the situation, it is obvious that growth of new technology only creates fear and apprehension among the youth. With some estimates suggesting that 80 per cent of the jobs will get automated over the coming decades, job markets are obviously under real threat.

I am not a pessimist. There is certainly scope for the youth to bridge the gap between their current education and the challenges being posed by the advancement in technology. But in that scenario too, those who are already off the block will breast the tape first. Today's competition demands that the youth, the corporate world and most importantly the government change their outlook towards education and training.

Nepal needs to take on the new challenge without losing a minute.

Learn How To Unlearn

June 2022

Whatever may be our age, many of us are haunted by romantic songs about love and heartbreaks. The pain of separation has to be experienced to be described. Wrenching away oneself from a fond past, which once used to be your present, can indeed be painful. Intimate memories remain engraved on the heart that bleeds.

The ups and downs in personal life are not too different from the travails in our corporate experience. The need to part ways from the past and venture on a new path is integral to life, on both personal and business fronts. One has to move on for sheer survival and much needed transformation.

Enter *unlearning*.

Unlike poetry, unlearning in the business and corporate world is not about merely forgetting the past. That will create a vacuum. Companies need to promote and learn new skills to keep up with the needs of a volatile business environment.

However, as the business and corporate world has come to realize over the past decade and a half since the emergence of unlearning, its execution is easier said than done. We have focused too long on the *learning* organization. Unlearning to carve out a new path has, therefore, become that much more difficult. Victims of heartbreaks know how tough it is to find a new purpose and way in the world.

Companies and their rank and file too tend to fall in love with their set ways over a period in time. They take pride in their work style. It is almost like age-old customs in different social groups. Any change or reform rattles the society and protest follows. Companies and their employees too are part of a social system and are wary of changes. So, the reaction to new things is likely to be the same. Herein the role of top management assumes significance.

The needs of a networked economy can be met only with exponential changes. Gradual and incremental changes cannot take you far. By the time you give up some old work habits and acquire new ones the *new* would have become obsolete. Hence the need for rapid change and distancing from mental models that have served well earlier, but are no longer adequately effective now. This does not mean abandoning all old skills, lock, stock and barrel; rather you have to pick and choose with discretion and add new skills and knowledge to your portfolio. Needless to say that this should become a regular process.

Among companies that broke limits and opted for exponential growth are the likes of Google, Apple, Uber, Netflix, Airbnb and Facebook—a cluster that is perhaps envied by the corporate world.

So, how can we facilitate unlearning?

The top management, particularly in family-run organizations, needs to recognize and display that the existing mental model is no longer effective. This will spur others in the organization to at least look into the deficiencies in the old system. They will no longer be afraid of abandoning the old practices. Rather they will become more curious about the new system and also offer suggestions, making the organization less hierarchical in terms of decision-making. This buy-in by the rank and file is the first step towards the success of unlearning.

After this, you should obviously create and present a business model that is better aligned to the realities faced by your company and the segment in which it is housed. Social media can play a vital role in this respect. It is not a mere channel for message distribution. Management experts advise that social media be viewed and used as a tool for communication from many to many; the one-to-many model of social media is falling apart.

Beware of the tendency of slipping back to the comfort zone of old practises viewed mostly among employees who have been with you for a long time. Usually they are most resistant to change. After all, starting things afresh is strenuous and distancing from the past is painful. The past, imperceptibly, becomes one's real psyche and persona, and giving it up hurts in more ways than one.

Management practitioners and researchers have figured out several unlearning facilitators like using collaborative language, prompting employees to adopt small but mind-set altering measures like switching off electric equipment, laptops, etc., changing locations and increasing diversity in teams to foster cross-fertilization of ideas among persons with different backgrounds and skill sets, encouraging child-like curiosity among employees, and providing constant hand-holding and course correction.

By following the above measures in earnest the management can minimize not only its own sense of loss, but also of its employees that may be caused by the abandoning of old and obsolete models. Present them a new love in return.

Your Saviour Lies Within

August 2022

Nobody knows you better than yourself. You are therefore, best equipped to dive deep into your being and ferret out your faults and weaknesses. You can mend yourself best and fastest. In the process, you can emerge stronger, overcome challenges and court success.

Ever since we gained our senses, we have tasted failures and successes, big or small. So we are familiar with both. But we are more used to rejoicing over our achievements and brushing off our setbacks.

The most experienced analyst may not be able to detect the behavioural and mental shortcomings that caused setbacks in different stages of your life and career. You are the first to identify them. Let us start from our school days. We know if we used to avoid arithmetic, numbers and sums like the plague. We also know if we used to rely mostly on rote learning—the hitherto cornerstone of our educational system. Neither is it a secret that many of us were no great fans of analytical thinking and out-of-the-box solutions. If we loved languages, stories, poems, music, dance, arts or sports, then that too was known to us. We were the first to identify our pluses and minuses while others, including parents and teachers, might not have had that clear a view of our likes, dislikes, abilities and proficiencies.

Many of our young business executives and managers might not have fully understood the full relevance and value of concepts like intelligence quotient (IQ), emotional quotient (EQ), spiritual quotient (SQ), curiosity quotient (CQ), adaptability quotient (AQ), multiple intelligences (MI), or VUCA (volatile, uncertain, complex and ambiguous) environment during their school and college days. But now with some years of professional experience under their belt, they do realize the link between these concepts and their day-to-day managerial functioning. The imagined picture in the mind takes shape. Bright budding managers realize the presence, absence, abundance or paucity of these quotients most intricately and vividly. It is up to them to fortify their professional arsenal, either themselves or with external help. But the first step involves acceptance of the weaknesses that you see within yourself. The ego may prompt you to go astray. But self-betrayal can lead to utter ruination of your corporate dream.

Upcoming managers are often bombarded with the clichéd saying: failures form the stepping stone to success. Yes it is true to some extent, but are we by implication suggesting that managers should smilingly invite failures and gloat over them once floored? That would be far from the truth.

By encouraging honest self-introspection by children and students from their earliest days we can prepare them against debacles and setbacks. The fire of failures scars and scorches grievously. The pain and agony linger for long. Would it not be better to prepare our children and youth to keep failures at bay as early as we can? I know we cannot rule out fiery setbacks in businesses but we can certainly minimize their occurrence and fight them better with a proactive attitude and approach.

This calls for what I describe as the 'quotient deficit management' for and by young managers with active and sustained help from the HR department and, if need be, external coaches. Regularly available mentors can be a great help in filling gaps in the above mentioned quotients and allied skills for successful execution of respective roles of upcoming managers. In view of increase in job rotation, the focus needs to be on promoting an amalgamation of quotients.

The top management must drive out the belief held by many young executives that failure is the end of the road. There are multiple reasons behind the collapse of a company or a project. No junior manager has ever pulled an enterprise single-handedly. However, failure, individual or corporate, pulverizes perception. Such enthusiastic but wet-behind-the-ears managers need to be convinced that guilt which is uncalled for, victimhood and persecution complex are not going to take them anywhere.

The ABC of Team Building

September 2022

Compared to a couple of decades ago, these are great times for young managers. The chances of being asked to build your own team and execute projects are far brighter now.

Young as you are, with a few years of experience you may feel nervous and intimidated and may even refuse to take up the challenge. But if you are a smart one, you will see it as an opportunity to move up the career ladder. You have to understand that the senior management has entrusted you with team-building responsibilities because it sees promise and potential in you.

What should you do to attain success in team building?

First, you must immediately realize and internalize the reality that henceforth your success will be measured by the success of your team and not by your personal accomplishments. You are no longer a solo player.

For this to happen, you must have an elaborate interaction with your reporting authority to clearly understand the organization's expectations from your team. This will enable you to choose members most suited for the forthcoming collaboration.

Having received an explanation about the objectives of the team by your superiors, you need to convey these expectations to each individual member of the team as well as to the team as a whole. Any vagueness or confusion at this stage may lead to the team members straying in different directions.

The best way to keep such risks at bay is to have a one-to-one meeting with each team member. Match and mix an individual's abilities and skills with the team's overall objectives. As the team leader, you need to be a highly attentive listener. Create a congenial atmosphere for the team member/s to open and articulate their strengths and weaknesses. This is for your own good as no leader is a master of all trades and needs support and advice from all their teammates. Even a single wrong selection by you may undo the entire team's efforts.

Your team selection process is still not complete. Focus on knowing what motivates the individual team members best as no two members' motivations may be the same. This input about specific team members will help you calibrate your HRD, behavioural and reward schemes (not necessarily monetary) accordingly to ensure optimal output from the entire team. You will notice that timely and public recognition of outstanding employees can boost their morale way higher than mere financial incentives. They are quick to realize how their achievements add to their learning and overall growth prospects. Companies value team builders and players.

As you move ahead with team building, you will also find that almost all employees want to excel in their areas and multiply their skill sets by collaborating with their other team members who have different talents and expertise. There are no born laggards and shirkers. A good team leader can transform even slow movers into agile and nimble performers.

But this is easier said than done. Once the team is put into place and it starts moving towards its clearly enunciated individual-specific and group goals, maintaining the momentum assumes great significance. This can be made possible if there are continuous and candid conversations between the team leader and the team members. The corporate world describes this as feedback.

I prefer the term two-way feedback and there is a reason for it. We witness mostly top-to-bottom flow of ideas and instructions for course correction in the developing world where hierarchy is still paramount in business and society. But it has often been seen that the most urgent pain points, as well as sweet spots, are first experienced by the employee engaged in a specific task. But the employee concerned does not share the matter with the leader or superior authority fearing adverse repercussions.

To bridge this trust deficit you will need to create an aura of psychological safety in your team to encourage its members to speak out. Many team leaders have been seen to falter on this front. Frank and regular discussions between the team leader and players are imperative. It has often been seen that feedback from the team leader and his players has prompted the top management to tweak its goals more in line with the existing business reality. It is not so uncommon to find the market scenario changing even as the team is working on a project. Old assumptions lose their relevance. The team usually discovers this much before the top management, but does not report, fearing reprimand and reprisal. Eventually, the company gets hit. Hence, the high value attached to regular two-way feedback.

Thankfully, comprehensive feedback is gradually becoming the norm in more and more companies, particularly in the advanced countries. The socio-cultural environment in our part of the world is a dampener in this respect. However, the disadvantages of sticking to archaic ways of business are far too many. I can see the resultant change happening.

Made in the USA
Monee, IL
13 May 2026

237f14d0-2f54-4305-8302-578a9103c8dcR01